# Praise for *Surviving Cancer*

This is an excellent book…very informative and useful. It is factually supported, eminently readable and lucidly written. *Surviving Cancer* provides insight and valuable advice for anyone who has been diagnosed with cancer. As an oncologist working in this field for decades, I highly recommend this book.

M.V. PILLAI. MD, FACP
PRESIDENT & CEO, INCTR(USA)
CLINICAL PROFESSOR OF ONCOLOGY
THOMAS JEFFERSON UNIVERSITY, PHILADELPHIA, PA
& SENIOR ADVISOR—GLOBAL VIRUS NETWORK (GVN.ORG)

Whether you're interested in preventing cancer or stopping its spread once it has been diagnosed, John M. Poothullil's book will be an invaluable resource. With dietary recommendations, thoughts on exercise and supplements, stress-related information, and more, the book is a complete guide for those who want to fight against cancer. A must-have for those at high risk of developing the disease, *Surviving Cancer* provides sound research and actionable steps that anyone can follow in order to live a longer and healthier life.

ANGELA WOLTMAN
FOREWORD MAGAZINE

*Surviving Cancer* offers several new perspectives on cancer that don't appear in other books, despite the volume of literature produced yearly about cancer survival. Readers willing to make lifestyle changes to prevent, limit, and curtail cancer's appearance and spread will find this book offers not just hope, but a proactive approach that places patients in charge of many different options.

D. DONOVAN
MIDWEST BOOK REVIEW

# Surviving Cancer

# SURVIVING CANCER

A New Perspective on Why Cancer Happens
& Your Key Strategies for a Healthy Life

**John M. Poothullil, MD, FRCP**

**Author of *Diabetes: The Real Cause and the Right Cure***

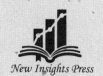

New Insights Press

Editorial Direction and Editing: Rick Benzel Creative Services, rickbenzel@msn.com
Book Design: Ryan Scheife, Mayfly Design
Cover Design: Susan Shankin
Text Illustrations: Kayla Benson, kabillustrations@gmail.com

Published by New Insights Press, Los Angeles, CA

First edition printed in the United States of America

Library of Congress Control Number: 2017913012

ISBN: (print) 978-0-9984850-2-7

ISBN: (eBook) 978-0-9984850-3-4

# IMPORTANT NOTICE

**THIS BOOK IS NOT INTENDED TO REPLACE THE CARE OF A PHYSICIAN.** It presents a new explanation on the causes of cancer and how you may be able to prevent it from spreading or re-occurring in the future. The recommendations provided can help a reader with cancer as well as those with cancer and high blood sugar or Type 2 diabetes. If you follow the recommendations, we suggest you work with your physician.

**THE DISCUSSIONS IN THIS BOOK CONCERNING DIABETES ARE RELEVANT ONLY FOR THOSE WHO HAVE TYPE 2 DIABETES. THE INFORMATION ABOUT TYPE 2 DIABETES IS NOT APPLICABLE TO TYPE 1 DIABETES,** in which the pancreas is damaged and does not produce enough insulin for the body to utilize sugar. Type 1 diabetes is a disease that usually strikes in childhood. Type 1 diabetes can be traced specifically to a lack of insulin production by the pancreas. If you have cancer and Type 1 diabetes, consult your doctor.

# Contents

## Part 2: How to Survive Cancer

## Part 3: Key Points and Conclusions

# Prologue

FEAR. FEAR IS WHAT MOST PEOPLE FEEL UPON RECEIVING A DIAGNOSIS OF cancer—and perhaps you are experiencing it. The capacity to feel fear is an integral part of human nature, but so are adaptations that allowed our ancestors to survive life-threatening situations for tens of thousands of years.

HOPE. Hope is my objective in writing this book, to share with you that it is possible for most people confronted with the prospect of dying from cancer to lessen the degree of threat that cancer makes on their life. There are real actions you can take to prevent yourself from dying from cancer. If reading this book reduces the intensity and duration of your cancer-related anxiety and fear, I will have accomplished my minimum objective in writing it.

In a nutshell, you will learn that if you have been diagnosed with a solitary cancer, such as a tumor, it may cause symptoms due to its location or size. But in a vast majority of cases, a solitary cancer can be treated, or removed. It is when that cancer releases thousands of cancer cells that roam all parts of the body, scouting for suitable locations to start their own housekeeping that makes cancer life threatening. If even just a few succeed, they can create enough disruption of metabolic processes in the body to endanger life itself. They do so by confiscating nutrients your normal cells need to sustain themselves, not just in one site but in multiple parts of your body.

As a metaphor, we have to think of cancer as an iceberg in the ocean and you are a boat approaching it. One can't know the true size of the iceberg by looking at the top of it. You can only see the portion above the water, and what is beneath the sea is far larger. Similarly, one can't know how long a cancer has been in existence when it is detected; it may have been growing for years, if not decades. One can navigate around a solitary iceberg once the location and the direction of the iceberg's movement is known. More often than not, one can survive a solitary cancer once the location and size are known. But the chance of an accident increases when one has to navigate around multiple icebergs. In the same way, when the number of cancers or cancer sites in the body is increased, the chance of survival is reduced.

My message is that many types of cancer are survivable—and this book will serve as your guide around the iceberg. In reading these pages, you will see that the body can continue living while accommodating a solitary cancer. There are actions you can take that may prevent it from spreading, even if there are complications. How to use this knowledge to face the threat and survive is the hopeful news you will get in these pages.

## The why of cancer

Cancer has been present throughout human history. Our 21st century science has come a long way in understanding cancer: how some cancers (but not all) are caused, how some cancers (but not all) may be successfully treated, and how some cancers (but not all) can be prevented from occurring or recurring in individuals. But, in general, the prevention and complete eradication of all cancers still eludes us.

This book is my contribution to the literature on cancer and reflects my decades of study as a trained MD. In my thinking about the human body and the causes of disease, my emphasis has been on cancer and diabetes. In these pages, I present new ideas and insights into what cancer fundamentally is, how it occurs in the body, why it is so hard to "cure," and what choices each of us has—individually and collectively—to prevent cancer-related death. My explanations for why cancer happens are extremely important to understand, especially if you have been diagnosed with it.

## Who this book can help

My objective in writing this book is to reduce the incidence of cancer-related deaths in general, but especially in four populations.

1. This book will be an invaluable resource for **anyone who has already been diagnosed with cancer** localized to a single site of origin and not yet colonized in another part of the body.

2. I also write this book for **anyone who believes they are at risk of cancer** due to heredity, lifestyle, working conditions, stress levels, or for any other reason. As you will see, my strategy for preventing death from cancer opens a new path to understanding it and being able to take actions to ensure it does not happen to you.

3. This book will be especially important for **anyone with Type 2 diabetes**, a population that is twice as likely to develop certain types of cancer compared to individuals who do not have diabetes. I became familiar with this statistic because I have been researching and studying Type 2 diabetes for more than 20 years. During this time, I developed new theories and ideas to explain how high blood sugar develops and becomes Type 2 diabetes. In 2015, I published a book, *Eat, Chew, Live*, to explain those concepts and teach people how to avoid Type 2 diabetes. In addition, in July 2017, I published *Diabetes—The Real Cause and The Right Cure: 8 Steps to Reverse Your Diabetes in 8 Weeks*, to help those who are already diagnosed with diabetes. Along my journey to understand high blood sugar and diabetes, I became especially intrigued as to why people with high blood sugar levels have a higher incidence of cancer than people who do not have high blood sugar. In applying my knowledge about the cause of Type 2 diabetes to the biology of cancer, I developed several insights that I believe help explain the link between diabetes and cancer.

4. Lastly, I also seek to help **anyone who is a survivor of cancer**, so you can better understand what you can do to live as long and as well as possible. Many cancer survivors succumb to the same or different cancer years after their first diagnosis and treatment, but it is possible to influence this outcome.

The diabetic audience for this book is a growing one. According to the International Diabetes Federation, in 2015 there were 415 million people living with diabetes in the world, and that number will climb to 642 million by the year 2040. Given that diabetes is considered a serious epidemic now, this statistic means that cancer is likely to follow and become the next epidemic as more and more diabetics develop it. The growth of cancer cases will impact the financial resources of both developed and developing countries, as well as the pocketbook of every individual who is affected. Therefore, another objective of this book is to describe a methodology to reduce the incidence of cancer in people who have high blood sugar, such as those diagnosed with prediabetes or diabetes. Understanding this will help you learn what to do to prevent cancer and how to do it.

Overall, my sincere hope is that the information in this book will help you and your loved ones—no matter which of the above groups you might belong to: newly diagnosed with cancer, healthy but concerned, diabetic, or a survivor of cancer. Your journey with me begins by understanding how cancer starts. We will then see how it survives and spreads, and how you can starve it so a single tumor or localized cancer site can be successfully treated without your unknowingly setting up the conditions that help cancer spread throughout the body.

I believe many people can do much to prevent or postpone the occurrence of cancer, halt a reoccurrence, or prevent its spread—so that you can be in charge of living a healthy life for as long as possible, experiencing what matters to you most.

## Overview of this book's insights

Just as it helps to have a map to plan your journey, it can help to understand in advance the points I will be making in this book. Here is an overview of the insights I will impart to you:

1. You may not know it, but during everyone's lifetime, cancer cells are continually formed in the body at various intervals as a result of various metabolic activities and environmental exposures. Changes to the genes in charge of cell multiplication are happening constantly, leading to the potential for the uncontrolled division of cells—and that is what cancer is. Such genetic change occurs even in people with no genetic predisposition to cancer. To put it bluntly, *cancer cells are a normal occurrence in every human being.*

2. Your immune system usually recognizes these wayward cells that are not functioning as they are supposed to. The immune system then sends out signals for those cells to self-destruct. Most of the time, this self-destruction occurs, but sometimes those initial cancer cells resist the signal and begin multiplying.

3. The deadly element of cancer arises when those cells continue to multiply and multiply. They then send out "daughter cells" to other parts of the body where they do the same. Soon the cancer cells take over space needed by normal cells, disrupting the functioning of bodily organs. Why do cancer cells do this? My insight here is that *multiplying is the primordial survival mechanism of any cell.* From the very first cell on Earth that divided into two so that it would have another cell, all its progeny cells survived when their own useful life was

over by multiplying. The fact is, *every cell with a nucleus is driven to divide*. No matter what other cellular operations do not function in them, all cells are pre-programmed to reproduce if they are alive. This is an important key to understanding cancer.

4. Since the primordial urge of a cell in the body is to multiply, there may be nothing we can do to prevent it. This means that we may never be able to "cure" the disease of cancer, technically speaking. What we can do, however, is to seek to limit the multiplying, as well as to prevent the cells in an initial cancerous site from spreading to other parts of the body.

5. All cells need energy to multiply, including cancer cells and their satellites. That energy comes from glucose. As you will learn, cancer cells are able to dominate other cells by grabbing the glucose in the fluids surrounding cells, thus fueling themselves more aggressively to multiply beyond the level that the body's immune system can handle. This is why people who have high blood sugar are at a greater risk of cancer than those whose blood sugar levels are normal.

6. High blood sugar, as well as some of the medicines that are used to treat it, causes the pancreas to produce more insulin, the hormone that helps glucose get into cells where it is used for cellular fuel. The conundrum is, insulin is a growth hormone and so high levels of insulin actually stimulate cells to divide, including cancer cells.

7. The combination of these two factors—glucose and insulin—effectively means that the more carbohydrates you eat, the more glucose in your bloodstream, and thus the greater the risk that you are stimulating the production of insulin. This brings on a "double whammy" for diabetics with cancer (and even for pre-diabetics, people with somewhat high blood sugar levels, but not high enough to be called diabetic). The higher levels of insulin in the body act as a stimulant for cancer cells to grow and multiply, while the glucose provides fuel for that reproduction.

8. Given the above insights, the best method to avoid the establishment of cancer, as well as prevent it from occurring in another part of the body or having it occur again after you have been treated for it, is to take these steps:

   a. Refrain from eating grains, grain-based products, and other high carbohydrate and sugar-laden foods in quantities that produce excess glucose in your bloodstream that will fuel cancer cells. You need to starve cancer cells to the greatest extent possible.

   b. Eat a diet of minimally processed vegetables, fruits, animal products, dairy, nuts, seeds, and fresh herbs and spices that will provide your body with the macro- and micro-nutrients your cells need to function optimally. Such a diet will also help nurture the beneficial bacteria in the gut that strengthen your immune system, which is your body's natural defense against cancer cells. The immune system is programmed to find and kill newly formed cancer cells, and so it must remain as strong as possible.

c.  At the same time, minimize your risks of introducing into your body foods containing agents that can damage your genes.

d.  Reconnect with your "authentic weight"—the weight your body is most comfortable at and which allows your blood sugar and insulin levels to stay in a normal range. Excess body fat is now recognized as a major contributing factor in America's cancer toll, ahead of tobacco.

e.  Exercise to condition your body and maintain your health, but do not count on exercise to lose weight.

f.  Avoid cancer-causing agents in the environment around you, as they have the potential to cause genetic mutations that may trigger cancer cells to begin forming, growing, and multiplying.

g.  Avoid exposure to infective agents such as human papilloma virus that can cause persistent infection, resulting in cancer. Keep in mind that HPV vaccines can prevent the infection in most cases if taken between the ages of 9 and 13. In addition, hepatitis B vaccine (HBV) is protective against liver cancer.

Some of you may consider cancer as a physical condition to be dealt with by medical professionals. For someone else, it is one's fate to endure. And for others, cancer is an incomprehensible and fearful affliction. No matter what you feel, you can take actions to survive. If the survival instinct of a cell makes cancer possible, as you will understand from reading this book, it is the same instinct in you that should prompt you to follow the precepts outlined.

## The unique format of this book

The rest of this book is divided into 3 Parts, organized logically so you can understand the causes of cancer, how it develops and possibly spreads in the body, the methods we currently have to detect it, and what you can do if you have been diagnosed with a cancer.

### Part 1—The Why of Cancer
- How Cancer Starts and Survives
- How Cancer Cells Grow
- How Cancer Spreads to Other Tissues and Organs (Metastasis)

### Part 2—How to Survive Cancer
- A Diet-Based Strategy to Starve Cancer Cells and Feed a Healthy Body
- Weight Control, Losing Fat, & Exercise
- Protecting Yourself Against Environmental Toxins & Pollutants
- Stress Management, Mindset, Sleep, and Hope

### Part 3—Summary of Key Points and Conclusion

# Divided into "paired pages"

Each of these sections, except for the Conclusion, contains many one-page essays. But I have organized these essays in a unique format, according to the level of scientific detail in each one.

- **LEFT-HAND PAGES** contain **basic information entries**. These are written in a very straightforward way, with only a modicum of scientific explanation for each idea. These pages are the main paths through the book. If you don't enjoy science, read only **these left-hand pages** and you will receive the essential information.

- **RIGHT-HAND PAGES** contain **more detailed and sometimes scientific entries**. These go much deeper into the science behind the concept on each prior left-hand page and are offered to you to read if you desire. Although some may be more challenging than others, not every one of them is difficult to understand, so give them a try.

I developed this format because I know many people find it hard to read scientific material. You may not have had biology class since you were in junior high school, or you find that science contains too much unfamiliar terminology. So I have constructed the book to contain these two types of entries to help you. I invite you to read each LEFT-hand page entry first, then, as you desire, read the corollary RIGHT-hand page that contains additional supporting scientific information.

But if you prefer to have just the basic information, you can read only the LEFT-hand pages of the entire book and look at the various illustrations and captions, even if they occur on a right-hand page. In this way you will learn all you need to know.

To understand and discuss cancer, there are times when learning the science behind the story is truly worth your effort, so I do hope you will, at some time, try to read the right-hand entries as well. The more you understand the biology behind how your body operates, the more

> **Read this left side for basic information. Then if you want more details, read the information on the facing right page.**
>
> **Read this right side for more details and scientific explanations, usually corresponding to the left-hand page.**

you will understand the rationale for changing your diet and doing everything you can to defeat your cancer and prevent it from reoccurring in the future. Most importantly, the information in each pair of entries combined will help you the most in understanding how to prevent the spread of cancer to other parts of the body. In short, knowledge helps you take charge of the health of your own body.

## Special section on grains

A critical theme in this book is that grains and grain-flour products are a major source of nutrition for cancer cells. For this reason, I have also written a special section that you will find in Part 2 about why you need to avoid eating grains if you have been diagnosed with cancer. This is especially important if you are also prediabetic or diabetic, as high blood sugar and cancer are highly linked.

# The Why of Cancer

In an evolutionary sense, mutations in a cell's genetic code create beneficial actions that usually help the survival of an organism. However, some mutations lead to cancer, which does not benefit an individual. So why do cells codify and pass cancerous mutations to the next generation of cells? This is the why of cancer we must understand.

# A new perspective on the why of cancer: The Adam Cell

For most people diagnosed with cancer, their first questions are, "How did I get this? Why me?" Let me try to answer you by introducing a completely new concept about cancer. This is a breakthrough theory that might give you profound insight into the cause of cancer—and why science may never be able to prevent it completely from happening.

Cancer is, as you know, the uncontrolled multiplication of cells. The body is made of billions of cells, with each organ or tissue composed of cells specialized to function according to what that tissue or organ is supposed to do. In other words, every cell has a job and is supposed to do that job to allow you to survive. Normal cells "behave" when they function and divide only when they are supposed to.

Cancer cells, however, do not behave as they are supposed to. Rather they divide and divide uncontrollably. They crowd out other cells in a site, incapacitating the normal cells surrounding them. And they may spread out throughout the body, taking over. Why do they do this?

As I gave thought to this over many years of study, I came to conclude that the only answer that makes any sense is that cells are, by default, driven to divide to survive. Perhaps billions of years ago, some cell on Earth, compelled to eat, drink, and defend itself, realized that it could continue living by dividing itself into two, rather than simply dying. I have called this cell "the Adam Cell," because it is the original ancestor of all cells that multiply. This Adam Cell endowed itself with the gift of immortality by codifying in its genes the ability to divide into two whenever it needed to survive. (It is likely that cells may have risen and divided in multiple locations on Earth. The Adam Cell is the embodiment of this fundamental concept.)

This same code is contained inside every one of the Adam Cell's progeny cells, to be used in tissue remodeling and wound healing later in life, if and when necessary. *This means that multiplication is an inherent capability in the early stages of every cell's existence.* We cannot stop the potential of a cell endowed with this code from dividing into two. In short, every cell starts its life existentially driven to divide and divide.

With this concept in mind, it changes how we must now understand the transformation of a normal cell in the body to one that is cancerous. This makes "curing cancer" a conundrum, as it may be impossible to prevent cells from multiplying, even when they are dysfunctional, as cancer cells are.

However, this theory can also help you understand what you can do to fight your cancer, including surviving it.

# More on the why of cancer: The immortal gene

What drove an Adam Cell to divide? My answer is as follows. Every cell in a living body, except red blood cells, contains a nucleus, inside which are genes carrying instructions for biological activities of the cell, including division. Without genes, a cell cannot divide.

Genes are composed of nucleic acids. Deoxyribonucleic acid (DNA) contains genetic instructions used in the development and functioning of the cell. Ribonucleic acid (RNA) functions in converting the genetic information from genes into the amino acid sequences of proteins. Life evolved billions of years ago from proteins interacting in various ways.

The genetic code in all living cells is the same, with relatively minor exceptions. For all practical purposes, all living things on Earth started life from copies of the same gene, having the same message. The drive to divide is thus a function of our genetic matter seeking to help the cell in which it is encased survive, to ensure its own immortality. The cell is the gene's protection, and for the gene to survive, the cell must multiply rather than die.

Fortunately for all life on earth, genes did more than simply cause a cell to divide—they also adapted. Living things evolved because genes accumulated changes that caused differences in messages coded in the genes. Each change led to some type of alteration in the shape of the proteins produced. The new shape enabled a protein to carry out different chemical reactions inside cells. These step-by-step alterations allowed specializations of cells as well as changes in the shape and size of cells, organs, and even the organism, making evolution possible.

In this way, allowing mutations appears to be the only way for genes, the masters of the cell, to ensure their own long-term survival. Imagine a group of cells exposed to a toxin it has never encountered before. The genes in charge of protecting the cells might be able to unleash enzymes to neutralize the toxin, but since the toxin is new to the cells, those enzymes would need to tweak their ability to repel it in different ways. In attempting to do this, most of the cells may die—but a few may survive. Survival of even one cell is enough to endow all the progeny cells with the same capability. In other words, survival was made possible by the innovative application of capabilities that already existed inside the cell.

## CURIOUS TIDBITS

As organisms evolved, cells seem to have decommissioned genes no longer needed for survival. However, cells had no mechanism to remove old genes and therefore continued to incorporate them in their newer models. This could be one of the reasons why when a chromosome is straightened out, it ranges in length from 3 miles to eighteen miles.

# Characteristics of a human cell

Human cells retain the capacity for independent life, before they are committed to be part of an organ or system in the body. Cells come in various shapes and sizes. Each cell contains proteins designed for specific tasks, and enzymes to assist in the metabolic activities needed for survival, whether as an individual cell or as part of an organism. A cell does not share components designed for inside work with its neighbors and keeps those components confined by a membrane. Although the membrane seals the cell, it allows specific molecules to pass to the inside from the environment outside, as well as going outside from the inside, after inspection by gatekeepers embedded in the membrane.

Trillions of cells compose your entire body—every piece of tissue and skin, all your bones, muscles and nerves, plus your arteries, veins, and blood, your entire brain matter, and all your internal organs. Each organ of your body is composed of hundreds of millions of independent cells, working together. The proper functioning of metabolic activities inside trillions of cells, and the coordination of working with others outside, are what maintain the health and well-being of a human being.

The inner body of the cell contains its command and control center, called the *nucleus*. The nucleus is in charge of issuing instructions for the construction of proteins that cells need to function. Inside the nucleus are twenty-three pairs of chromosomes, each one having long strands of genes that contain instructions for all activities the cell performs.

Outside the nucleus, each cell contains multiple small units, like little factories—some stationary and some mobile—called *organelles*, which function independently. Each has gatekeepers in charge of allowing the entry and exit of materials in and out of its membrane. Materials are transported between organelles on thin filaments that serve as roadways, sometimes using *vesicles*, similar, in our factory analogy, to little trucks.

One special type of organelle is called the *mitochondrion*. This is where a cell produces a lot of its energy in the form of ATP, which stands for *adenosine triphosphate*, the chemical cells use to power their functions. A cell has many mitochondrion (plural: mitochondria).

Note: The vast majority of cancer cells do not have functioning mitochondria. This is an important clue in preventing the growth and spread of cancer, as we will soon discuss.

# Pondering cells on Earth

You might be asking, where did the very first cell come from? What originated life on Earth? Without regard to any religious philosophy, the scientific answer to this question is that organic matter has existed on this planet for about 4 billion years. Beyond that, science has never really been able to answer the question.

The seventeenth-century English scientist Robert Hooke saw vacant chambers, similar to rooms occupied by monks, in a slice of cork under the microscope, and called them cells. Yet until the mid-nineteenth century, it was universally believed that life came on this earth only as whole organisms, whether animal, bird, or human being.

Now it is well known that atoms and molecules, when put into the right environment, can link together into predictable arrangements without external forces or guidance, because of their innate propensity for organization, called "self-assembly." A mathematically predictable and precise example is the crystallization of water forming ice in the kitchen refrigerator, with bonds between adjacent oxygen and hydrogen atoms in molecules of water. Even though the bonds between the atoms are weak, they are critical to controlling the structure and behavior of both water and ice.

The concept of self-assembly applied to molecules of protein can explain the origins of the architecturally complex living unit of a cell. Inside a cell, all fundamental chemical reactions needed for survival happen in a fluid medium. Membranes wall off the compartments, called organelles, designed for a specific function with motorized modules, called vesicles, moving materials and products on pre-established pathways in between.

It is only the living cell that can duplicate itself, among all the objects in the known universe. Although a lone cell ceases to exist upon death, if it has divided, survival of one of its duplicates effectively means survival of the same cell.

Shinya Inoué, a biophysicist and cell biologist and a member of the National Academy of Sciences, suggests, "Cell division is one of the great mysteries of life."

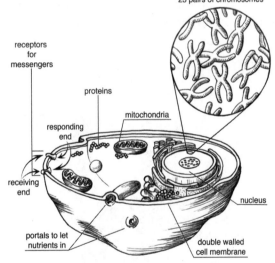

Labels: 23 pairs of chromosomes; receptors for messengers; proteins; mitochondria; responding end; receiving end; nucleus; portals to let nutrients in; double walled cell membrane

Every cell has a membrane that surrounds it and defines its boundary. On each cell membrane, there are specific proteins that identify what organ or tissue the cell is part of. The cell membrane is resistant to the unwanted entry of fluids (like water) that surround the cell, but it has portals where materials can enter and cell products and waste can exit. The portals are told to open or close in response to specific commands from the nucleus sent to the location. Every cell membrane also has receptors for receiving messages from hormones, other molecules, chemicals, and nerves.

# Chromosomes and genes: Drivers of cell reproduction and functionality

All cells in the body contain the same 23 pairs of chromosomes. They are in pairs because we inherit a copy of each chromosome from each of our parents.

Genes determine the inheritance of our biological characteristics, both good and bad, from our parents. It takes multiple genes to determine most of our biologic traits—e.g., our eye, skin, and hair color; our bone structure; our mental capacities; and so on. The combination of genes for each trait acts like a backup system; if one gene is incapacitated, others may be able to compensate for it.

Of the perhaps 25,000 genes in a human cell, only a fraction of them are active at any given time, based on the cell's metabolic needs. The activation of selected genes determines what functions each cell performs at any given time in producing proteins. Each protein has a different purpose and needs to get attached to a specific site within the cell that recognizes its configuration. Once attached, it starts a cascade of metabolic activities. Genes in charge of housekeeping activities are active on a more or less constant basis, while most other genes operate sporadically.

As you probably know, defective genes can cause cells to go haywire, leading to cancer. For this reason, it's critical to understand chromosomes and genes.

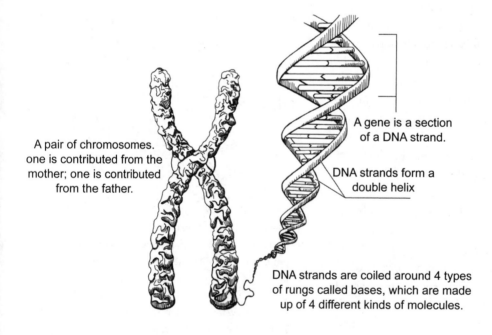

A pair of chromosomes. one is contributed from the mother; one is contributed from the father.

A gene is a section of a DNA strand.

DNA strands form a double helix

DNA strands are coiled around 4 types of rungs called bases, which are made up of 4 different kinds of molecules.

A pair of chromosomes, forming an X shape. Each chromosome contains thousands of genes, with each gene made of interconnected strands of DNA.

# How genes control the function of cells

The DNA in genes contains the recipes for each and every protein a cell is capable of making. There are almost a million proteins in the body, each one a little different. Proteins can't be formed without DNA, and only DNA has the recipe that can produce proteins. In order for both to happen, a cell is needed.

In other words, by themselves proteins and DNA can't accomplish anything—they need the protective environment inside a cell to carry out the function they are made for. If newly formed proteins do not pass inspection, both structural and functional, they are dismantled and their components reused—a sort of recycling at the cellular level.

To start an activity, genes send instructions for various enzymes residing outside of the nucleus through messengers made of Ribonucleic acids (microRNA). When the level of the product the enzymes are making reaches a threshold, their further action is inhibited. This precisely programmed, constant, planned activity allows all cells to live in their environment, contributing to the well-being of the entire body.

### CURIOUS TIDBITS

- Human genes contain recipes not only for producing proteins used by humans but also for those used by lower animals. For example, we carry genes capable of producing an animal part such as a tail, if it were activated by signals. (In 2016, a newspaper in India reported that an 18-year-old boy had an eight-inch tail removed; the parents as well as the child had hidden the fact of the tail until it had become too difficult for the boy to sit properly without experiencing pain.)[1] Inside a mother's womb, a baby has webbed feet or hands just as in duck feet. However, between the 6th and 7th weeks of pregnancy these webs are removed when genes responsible for producing them are deactivated and those responsible for fine-tuning fingers and toes become active.

- Genes in the nuclei of all cells in the body come from both parents. However, the genes responsible for controlling the mitochondria—the energy power plants of a cell—come from the mother, with rare exceptions.[2] This means that the survival of every cell in the body, and by extension the very existence of the human race, is made possible by energy produced by power stations designed by females!

# Cells have evolved to work together collaboratively, but cancer cells do not

Cells are equipped to live independently, meaning that each cell is able to meet all its internal needs to sustain life all on its own. This capability is accomplished through a variety of mechanisms inside the cell. There are mechanisms:

- to detect nutrients outside the cell
- to control the entry of those nutrients into the cell and use them
- to release material manufactured inside the cell and the waste products and heat made during daily life

As the cell consumes nutrients, it manufactures the products needed to sustain its life, by combining or dismantling the molecules of nutrients and other materials, and producing energy necessary for its functioning and reproduction.

Despite this capability to be independent, cells are programmed to live collaboratively with other cells, i.e., to be part of a larger organ or tissue. This means that individual cells living in groups must abide by rules that are important for the cohesive working of the group. Those that cannot do this are usually reprogrammed or destroyed.

What could have prompted cells to evolve to live together in groups? The most important reason might have been that forming groups helps maintain the ideal temperature for growth and reproduction. Individually, each cell has to spend some amount of its available fuel on a continual basis just to regulate its internal temperature, while losing some of the heat to the outside. But formed into a group, some of the heat coming out of one cell can benefit its neighbors.

This advantage of sharing heat may have started cells into forming groups. Perhaps by chance, a group of cells discovered the efficiency of heat retention by having a cover designed over the whole group—skin—in addition to the membranes enveloping each cell. This then led to other shared biological functions that are mutually beneficial, such as finding food. This may have then evolved into a point of specialization in which cells have separately defined functions among organ systems. In so doing, each cell becomes willing to voluntarily deactivate its capacity to function independently so it can live cooperatively with others.

As you might expect, cancer cells are different, as they do not respect the rules of neighborliness and collaboration.

# How cells form collaborative groups in organs and tissue

How does the body ensure that embryonic cells assigned to form an organ produce only the required number of cells and fit them in the right orientation relative to their neighbors and the boundary of the organ? The answer seems to be that cells work collaboratively in their unit to know what to do.

For example, while each embryonic cell has an unlimited capacity to multiply, repeated parts such as teeth are not fashioned by the action of individual genes. There is no gene for your incisor tooth, another for premolar, or a third for your molar.

Rather, the process starts with genes instructing cells to produce a bud of enamel at each of the sites where a tooth is to be located. The shape and size of each tooth are then guided by signals coming from cells surrounding the enamel bud. As the process continues, some of the neighborhood cells release inhibitor signals to limit the size of each tooth. In other words, various aspects of the construction are choreographed by signals from the surrounding environment.

This same pattern of signal interaction between buds and neighborhood cells is seen in the development of all our other organs. This means that each cell has to abide by instructions to be a "good neighbor" by maintaining a firm attachment to its neighbors and act according to the rules of the tissue it is part of. By this I mean cells have to respect the neighbors' space, share nutrients with them, and help with disposal of waste and excess heat.

Also, when embryonic cells reach their destination, such as the site of an organ like the heart, kidney, or skin, they forsake forever the ability to move again by deactivating genes that made their movement possible.

The only exceptions to this are cells where mobility is a prerequisite for function. For example, cells that specialize in surveillance retain the capacity to move in the locality they live, in order to detect invaders. Others, like red blood cells, are born to be on the move constantly. Another example is immune system cells that are sent to fight infection in different locations throughout the body. In addition to keeping their ability to move, immune cells also develop the capability to navigate different pathways in the body and to survive in unfamiliar neighborhoods and protect themselves. They also learn to understand the instructions to locate and identify the enemy, and do their job.

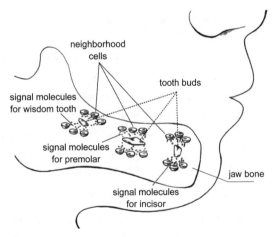

There is no gene that determines size and shape of each tooth. Rather, the process starts with genes instructing cells to produce a bud of enamel at each of the sites where a tooth is to be located. The shape and size of each tooth are then guided by signals coming from cells surrounding the enamel bud.

# How do cells get their energy?

It is important to understand how cells get their energy, as this plays a key role in cancer formation—and possibly in how we can prevent cancer.

As mentioned, the powerhouse in each human cell is the mitochondrion. This structure utilizes *either glucose or fatty acids* from the foods you eat, and converts them to energy molecules called *adenosine triphosphate*, ATP. But ATP can also be created outside the mitochondria using only glucose, though the production is not as efficient as inside the mitochondria.

Each cell in the body can manufacture ATP, and cells are constantly manufacturing it.

What does ATP do? ATP is like the batteries of a flashlight, available to power your body when it needs to implement any cellular process. (Virtually all cells in all organisms on earth produce and store energy needed for metabolic functions as ATP. ) ATP powers the production of protein molecules from raw materials. Like any manufacturing process, this takes energy. The cells of the body that use the most amount of ATP are in your skeletal muscles.

One of the most pivotal clues to stopping the growth of cancer is the fact that cancer cells in general do not have functioning mitochondria, even though some may have the structure.[3] Without mitochondrial actions, cancer cells are restricted to using only glucose to produce their energy outside the mitochondria, rather than being able to use both glucose and fatty acids inside them.

Do you see the importance of this? If you want to prevent cancer cells from multiplying, it might be useful to prevent them from getting glucose, right? I will reveal more about this shortly. Keep reading.

## CURIOUS TIDBITS

- The mitochondria were not part of the original cell design, but was a later evolutionary addition when the need to produce energy exceeded the basic process using glucose only. Mitochondria allowed cells to produce energy from a secondary source, fatty acids. Between meals, or when you exercise hard, your body will release fatty acids that have been stored in your fat cells to use as "backup" fuel. Having this secondary fuel source allows the liver to keep some glucose, which is released slowly into the bloodstream so as not to starve brain cells that preferentially use glucose rather than fatty acids as fuel.

- The enzyme that produces ATP and its underlying gene are very similar in all forms of life. In the process of photosynthesis, energy from sunlight is converted by plants to produce ATP that is used for the production of carbohydrates such as glucose. The most visible example of the use of ATP in metabolic activity is the conversion of chemical energy to particles of light by the firefly.

# The chemistry of cellular fuel: ATP

Cells are constantly making ATP. Millions of ATP molecules float around in each cell, ready to unload energy. Within ATP, energy is stored in the form of electrons, just as that coming through electric lines in your home, and can be used in the same fashion as you do when you flip a switch on.

The energy created from the decomposition of ATP is used for the metabolic reactions each cell is programmed to do. For example, ATP energy is used to link amino acids together to form protein molecules that are used to synthesize substances your body needs, such as hormones.

An individual, at any one time, has less than 10 oz. of ATP within all its cells combined because most ATP molecules are used up within two minutes after being made. But some remain unused, ready to be activated when your body needs energy at another time. All in all, each day the body produces enough ATP to equal its own body weight.[4]

However, the continual production of ATP without its corresponding usage is a wasteful process. Nature seems to have attempted to reduce this risk by a natural mechanism: when there starts to be an excess of ATP molecules, cells slow down their production.

### ⫸ CURIOUS TIDBITS ⫷

Nature took care of a potential conundrum—where to get the energy to make new cells before they have an existing mitochondrion. It turns out that when new cells are forming, the extraction of energy from glucose yields about 5% of the potential ATP energy that could be extracted from it. But this amount appears to be adequate to at least power the formation of the new cell's internal structures. Once the new cell has created its mitochondria, a full 100% of the potential energy from glucose can be extracted and made into ATP.

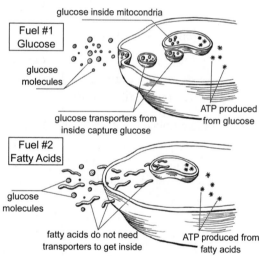

Fuel #1 Glucose

glucose inside mitocondria

glucose molecules

glucose transporters from inside capture glucose

ATP produced from glucose

Fuel #2 Fatty Acids

glucose molecules

fatty acids do not need transporters to get inside

ATP produced from fatty acids

Cells are like a hybrid car. They can use glucose to produce their energy, or they can use fatty acids to produce their energy. Note, however, that glucose needs "transporters" to get into a cell, but fatty acids can slip in without transporters, because the cell membrane is made of fatty acid and cholesterol molecules.

# Cell multiplication in normal cells is orderly

Cell multiplication in humans starts with conception, whereby a woman's egg cell splits into two cells within 24 hours after being penetrated by a sperm. This first division takes about 10 hours to be completed. Within the next 24 hours, those two cells split again, and then again. Those "embryonic cells" keep multiplying until billions of them with identical genetic material are formed.

We might compare it to someone having to build a second house identical to a first, reproducing precisely all rooms, appliances, plumbing, wiring and other amenities on site. The process starts with copying the instructions for building the house and everything in it and following the exact same process of construction as before.

From the very first division onward, every cell has the innate ability to divide and multiply itself. Even cells that have been kept in deep freeze for decades, when thawed and put in the right conditions in a laboratory, not only come back to life but also divide. Scientists all over the world use these cells to study normal biological mechanisms and to conquer diseases.

To understand cancer, it is important to know these two facts about cell multiplication:

- Every cell has a pair of *growth-activating* genes in charge of cell division. Activating one gene in a pair is enough to start the cell multiplication process.

- But every cell also has a pair of *growth-inhibiting* genes (also known as tumor suppressor genes) to stop cell division. Activating just one of these genes is enough to accomplish the objective.

This combination of activator/inhibitor signals is a common mechanism in many biological systems. The growth inhibitor acts as a sort of "fuse box" to cut off growth when the time is right.

As you might suspect, something goes awry with *both* growth inhibitor genes in cancer cells, which is why they keep multiplying. This is yet another clue as to what we need to learn about.

# The biology of cell multiplication and genes

The duplication of a cell is an orderly, designed process meant to maximize the functional groupings of cells. Each gene involved has to be activated in the right sequence to achieve the desired result.

It starts with an instruction to expose the gene containing the recipe. Once the gene is open, its internal machinery makes copies of all instructions related to the division of one cell into two, so that the new cell contains all the same instructions for further duplication with the potential for repeating the process.

A regulatory region, a tightly packed form of genetic material found just inside the wall of the cell nucleus, controls the function of the gene. This region contains ribonucleic acids called microRNAs that direct genes to allow the copying of instructions carried in them to create specific cells. The microRNAs also set a limit to the number of new cells by releasing regulatory messengers also made of RNAs.

Ordinarily, when normal cells die due to an infection or an outside agent that kills them off, the tissue they are part of is equipped with the capacity to regenerate new cells by activating already existing stem cells (the early stage of cells, as explained shortly) to begin reproducing, or by dividing existing normal cells. (In chronic diseases affecting an organ such as the kidney, this ability to regenerate new cells may be permanently lost.)

Since the stimulus to divide normally has to come from outside the cell, it is possible that dying cells may release protein messengers that are picked up by normal cells to tell them to start the process of cell division. This instruction must also tell cells to match, not overshoot, the target number of cells that are needed to bring the tissue back to a reasonable functional capacity.

The termination of cell multiplication can also happen in response to signals from neighboring cells, telling the cells that there is no more space.

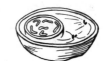

1) 23 pairs of chromosomes in nucleus

2) chromosomes replicate themselves

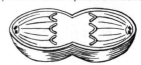

3) cell begins dividing; chromosomes split into two sets, one for each cell

4) 2 cells now exist, each with 23 pairs of chromosomes in the nucleus

A cell splits in an orderly fashion in a 4-step process, shown above.

# Phases of new cell development

In general, there are three phases during cell development:

- Phase 1 *embryonic stem cell*. These could become part of any tissue or organ, to be assigned by a master controller. In other words, any brand new cell could become a cell in any organ of the body at this time.

- Phase 2 *committed stem cells*. The embryonic cell changes to one that is designated to join a specific organ or tissue, but it is not yet assigned to a specified subgroup or task in the organ or tissue.

- Phase 3 *mature, fully differentiated cells*. These are cells that are functioning in their specific tissue or organ to do a specific task.

The transition from Phase 1 to Phase 2 occurs when a newly formed cell in the embryonic phase is directed to join one or another group of organs and tissues. This transition is achieved by taking away the ability to activate genes not needed for functioning in that organ or tissue. For example, certain genes in cells that will become the heart will be deactivated so the cell is unable to divide like normal cells, even when a signal for multiplication is outside its membrane. And while muscle cells can activate genes that produce "transporter" molecules that ferry glucose only *into* the cell, the liver can activate genes capable of producing transport molecules that move glucose *both in and out* of its cells.

To understand cancer, an important clue is that a new normal cell can become a cancer cell at any time during its development.

**CURIOUS TIDBITS**

When cells commit themselves to specific organs or tissues, some are asked to forgo the ability to multiply at a particular stage in their life. Without this ability to replace cells that die because of old age or injury, the very existence of the organism could be threatened. That is why most organs keep a supply of stem cells, one of which could multiply and quickly develop similar characteristics of cells that died, leaving a few stem cells behind for later use.

# Why stem cell research is valuable to help us understand cancer

In humans, a fertilized egg divides into cells, each one capable of multiplying to produce any type of cell in the body, or even a complete human being. These are called *embryonic stem cells*.

In the next stage of life for embryonic stem cells, the cells shut down many genes while keeping active those needed to become participants to form a particular tissue or organ. These are called *committed stem cells*.

Later, these cells deactivate even more genes while keeping active only those capable of tasks needed to be part of a tissue or organ. These are *mature, fully differentiated cells* with fixed identities.

Understanding the potential and limitations of embryonic stem cells to regenerate, and the capability (or not) of a cell with fixed identity to be reprogrammed to take on the characteristics of an embryonic stem cell, gives us both an opportunity to study normal mechanisms of cell division and also ways to control diseases like cancer.

For this reason, it is vital that we have cultures of human embryonic stem cells that allow us to use specific cell lines for research. One of the best examples of using this type of knowledge is research that led to the incorporation of stem cells into the body of a Type 1 diabetic, after which those stem cells began to function in the pancreas to produce insulin, which the Type 1 diabetic's pancreas had been unable to do before. (There are still problems such as rejection of implanted cells by the recipient's immune system, similar to what happened to cause the illness in the first place.)

# The body's normal mechanism for destroying abnormal and dysfunctional cells

In general, the body is vigilant in ensuring that you have healthy cells. It's normal for some cells to wear out and die on a regular basis. This timing can vary, depending on the organ. Skin cells may last for just a month, but cells in the liver can live for a few years, and nerve cells last a lifetime. Since every organ has the capability to replace worn-out cells, a process that goes on continuously, it is estimated that most of your body is reborn at the cellular level about every ten years.

Regardless of their natural lifespan, however, cells can suffer premature dysfunction, injury, or infection. Their death will then be initiated by signals from the inside or from other cells outside. For example, if a cell becomes dysfunctional, for whatever reason, it carries instructions within it to self-destruct. This is called *apoptosis*.

Programmed cell death can start even in the embryo stage. A cell suspected of being infected with a virus is instructed to die before completion of the cell's maturation cycle, to prevent the spread of the virus to nearby cells.

In addition, the body also seeks to eliminate cells that do not exhibit the ability to produce the normal amount of energy from glucose, or sources other than glucose. This is effectively an insurance program, because the amount of glucose needed to produce energy for a fully functional cell may not be always available in the fluid outside the cell. Cells must thus be able to produce energy from other fuels. As mentioned earlier, this is accomplished in the mitochondria, where not only glucose but also fatty acid components can be inserted into the energy extraction line whenever they are available.

If dysfunctional cells do not self-destruct, immune cells can also detect and cause the destruction of infected cells in the body. Immune cells roam around every part of the body looking for intruders such as bacteria, which they can identify by proteins on cell membranes. If something is found, the information is relayed to the regional lymph node that will produce new immune cells with specific capability to destroy the intruders. This is also a type of coordinated attack that can happen to destroy an enlarging colony of cancer cells.

In addition, the body has a special group called Natural Killer cells—NK cells—with the ability to detect and destroy cells that are stressed by energy need/production mismatch. In every individual, millions of such killer cells roam the body to detect and destroy cells that do not actively contribute to the welfare of the whole.

# The importance of cell self-destruction (*apoptosis*)

With trillions of cells in the body, and given that most cells reproduce very frequently, one might expect cellular damage to happen frequently—and it does. It is estimated that between 50 and 70 billion cells die each day in the average adult, and half that amount in an average child between the ages of 10 and 15.

There can be changes in cell structure and internal elements, such as genes, due to environmental agents that enter the cell, like viruses or asbestos. But other changes can be random mistakes. Therefore, there has to be a mechanism to get rid of unnecessary, damaged, or infected cells.

As a result, the body has to be vigilant to rid itself of defective and abnormal individual cells that can lead to uncontrolled multiplication and the potential for cancer formation. For example, if the cell receives a message from the neighboring cell about signs of unnatural intrusion into its environment, the nucleus will activate regulator mechanisms to curtail such activity. In addition, any critical damage to the genes of a new cell during its formation calls for its repair or removal.

One way this happens is that there are other genes that monitor cellular activity. If unnecessary or unexpected cellular functions are detected, the *growth-inhibiting* genes send out signal molecules, attempting first to save the cell, or if that fails, by triggering the programmed death of defective cells.

A second way unwanted cells are detected and repaired or removed is that the body's immune system monitors protein markers on cell membranes for clues of changes, or to detect invaders such as bacteria, viruses, parasites, and fungi. This biological tactic is similar to inspecting an employee's official entry badge in an office building, looking for signs of fraud. The immune cells can detect any changes that look unusual or different from what is expected in that cell. This allows the immune system to detect the entry of an alien, such as bacteria, and then mobilize to eliminate the cell before it can multiply to produce an infection.

Just as you incur expenses to dismantle an existing house, you incur energy expenditure to deconstruct an existing cell. Keeping the mitochondria active to produce the needed ATP until the last possible moment is how the body helps this important biological activity.

# Understanding adaptations and mutations

ADAPTATIONS ALLOW AN ORGANISM TO SURVIVE IN A NEW OR adverse environment. Cells, like people, require multiple nutrients for proper functioning. Nutrients have to be acquired from outside the organism, but that external environment is constantly changing. For example, regardless of where you live, the physical environment around you changes from day to day, and the nutrient environment changes from season to season. Both may even change from year to year.

In order to survive, the organism has to be prepared to face challenges that are unpredictable. Creating an environment for beneficial responses at the cellular level by changing the genetic instructions is what adaptations are all about. In general, most adaptations are for immediate usage under temporary conditions and for temporary purposes.

But the body has other physiological mechanisms if the challenge is long-term. After a long period of using adaptive mechanisms and understanding the benefit of them for successive generations, the organism may decide to make it permanent through gene mutations. A mutation is any change to cell genes so they function differently. Mutations are the fundamental basis of evolution.

Mutation is the only way a cell can pass on an adaptive capability needed for survival to the next generation. When organisms can't adapt, mutate, and pass the mutation to the next generation, they simply become extinct from nature.

The problem is that mutations of genes are also the foundation for a normal cell to acquire the capability to become a cancer cell.

# Cells can undergo mutations in their genes, but it is not always cancer

In addition to adaptations that lead to mutations, cells can also suffer damage to their genes that cause a mutation. Such mutations happen all the time, and most do not lead to cells becoming cancerous.

Here is an analogy. Each cell manufactures an estimated 2000 new protein molecules per second. Imagine a cell is like a busy sports arena with numerous chaotic activities all going simultaneously. On the field (the interior of the cell), professional teams are all playing different games (functions) at the same time: soccer, football, and rugby, for example. Each game is played by its own rules. Meanwhile, league officials are in the middle of the field (the cell nucleus with genes), protected by a thin wall. Their job is to issue instructions when messengers come in from referees and umpires on the field. On the field, players are constantly bumping into each other, and some get injured and need to be taken away. Designated workers remove damaged balls and equipment; field turf is repaired as needed; water and oxygen are brought onto the field when required. Meanwhile, play continues 24/7/365 with no time outs or stoppages.

In this chaos, genes can be damaged or altered, creating mutations. Mutations can take many forms, from a small change in the sequence of amino acids that make up the DNA inside the gene, to the complete absence of a particular gene. Or the mutation can also cause an extra gene to form, such as with Down syndrome. Of the many thousands of alterations experienced by genes, fewer than 1 in 1000 become permanent.

A cell can sustain itself even with only 20% of the original genes working. This means that mutations in most genes have little impact on the function of a cell. However, when a mutation in a gene is not repaired, it could be transmitted to successive cell generations and become permanent in all the further multiplications of those cells. It has been estimated that each human generation of people passes as many as 10 or more mutations on to its next generation.

But only a very small fraction of mutations ever lead to cancer, even with many trillions of new cells forming in a human body year after year.

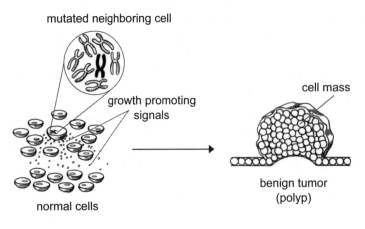

mutated neighboring cell

growth promoting signals

normal cells

cell mass

benign tumor (polyp)

Some people develop what is called a benign tumor—polyp, for example—that is a cell growing into a mass of tissue. A mutated gene in a cell sends out growth signals, causing neighboring cells to multiply. However, there is no mutation of genes among the multiplying cells or invasion of neighboring organs. Unlike cancer, benign tumors remain localized.

# The chemistry of how gene mutations happen

It is estimated that with all the activities going on inside a cell, each strand of DNA that is used to create a gene is attacked thousands of times every day by chemicals or protein molecules. In addition to injuries from physical contact, DNA injuries can also be produced by high-energy particles such as oxygen radicals created during metabolic activities inside the cell, as well as by ionizing radiation passing through the cell.

All in all, in a person's lifetime, each gene suffers millions of injuries. Most of these wounds are repaired swiftly, and do not have consequences on the cell function, especially if the repair is completed fast enough, or the affected protein still functions similarly with a different amino acid in place.

There is an elaborate set of gene repair mechanisms present in every living cell. And while the worker enzymes repair one strand of DNA, there is another strand of DNA containing the same information that still functions. This is the advantage of having chromosomes in pairs: one acts as a backup for the other in case a gene is damaged.

However, if the repair work is not completed before the cell divides, the mutated genes are divided in that form. Each daughter cell is then born with the mutated gene, and passes the same mutation on to the next generation of cells. This can result in diseases such as sickle cell anemia, muscular dystrophy, cystic fibrosis, and many others. The importance of DNA repair in uncontrolled cell multiplication is also evident in a medical condition called *xeroderma pigmentosum*. People who have this condition inherit a defective gene that results in incomplete repair work on skin cells damaged by ultraviolet radiation. They suffer a high rate of skin cancer.

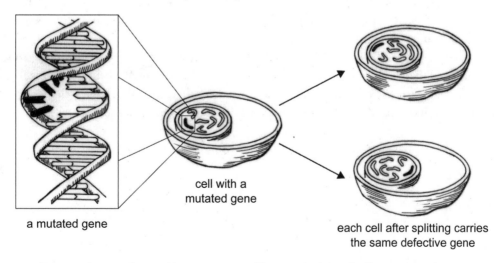

a mutated gene

cell with a
mutated gene

each cell after splitting carries
the same defective gene

Genes can become damaged for many reasons. The mutation in a cell will appear in each new cell after multiplication.

# Mutations are actually for benefit, but some end up as cancer

Why do cells even allow mutations to occur in the first place, and why do they let these cells live on, rather than ensuring that those cells self-destruct? I suggest that the answer has to do with my Adam Cell theory and the fact that life evolves, constantly seeking improvements.

Without mutations, cells can't adapt to a changing environment and the organism could become extinct. Beneficial adaptations codified as mutations are probably responsible for the progressive evolution of unicellular organisms into the eventual appearance of humans on this earth. This process took hundreds of millions of years and occurred step by step, as mutations in unicellular organisms resulted in the appearance of multicellular organisms. As suggested earlier, a multicellular organism may have started as a harmless group of cells that benefitted from each other and learned to ignore the established rules of separation.

Imagine how, to the unicellular organisms in the neighborhood, the multicellular organism may have been the equivalent of a cancer formation, depriving them of nutrients needed to grow. Yet they found no reason to attack this organism, or tumor, because it was in no way threatening their own existence. And as we said, the release of heat from the glob of cells may have benefitted unicellular organisms in the neighborhood. This is not unlike the tolerance shown by the human body to the presence of bacteria that outnumber our body cells by about ten to one, not only without threatening the body cells, but also providing benefits to the body, such as producing nutrients the body can use.

In effect, from an evolutionary point of view, it makes sense that nature allows cells to tolerate mutations. Cells are programmed from the Adam Cell to allow this freedom and flexibility, knowing that adaptation is the key to survival. While not really looking for it, a cell suddenly discovers the faculty to keep multiplying and comes to enjoy it, repeating the act at every available opportunity.

What is unclear, however, is why the body doesn't trigger the programmed death of any mutated cell that does not contribute to survival. It could be that even when the body is able to kill cells that are mutated, it simply cannot stop cells from dividing—the Adam Cell theory—no matter how dysfunctional, and those that escape destruction become cancerous cells.

# Mutations help organisms survive

After Charles Darwin formulated the idea that genetic mutations allowed species to evolve, a central dogma of biology took hold: that mutations that actually improve an organism's ability to survive in an environment are unpredictable. However, it has since been found that animal breeding in captivity to improve chances of survival can cause mutations that prove to be advantageous in animals, such as fish. But there is a price to pay: when they are released back into the wild, they may not survive as well compared to their ancestors because of the irreversible nature of mutations.

This confirms however, that beneficial mutations are those that help an organism survive *in its environment*. Some genetic mutations might happen this way. When a particular activity proves to be beneficial for an organism, it is codified and passed on to the next generation through a gene mutation.

An example of this is how we ended up with many different hormones that are structurally very similar but in charge of different and sometimes varied biological functions. The story might be that eons ago, a single hormone produced under the direction of a single gene carried out all functions. But as the organism evolved, mutations led to changes in the coding, resulting in two different hormones being produced with similar structure but more targeted functions.

For example, the two hormones *prolactin* and *growth hormone* have very similar amino acid sequences, and similar cells in the same location in the brain produce both hormones. But the two hormones differ in their function. Prolactin influences metabolic activities involved in the development of organs, blood vessels, blood cells, immune system, milk production, and a few other biological processes. Meanwhile, growth hormone is in charge of height, bone density, muscle mass, cell reproduction, and a few others.

It may be that this mutation stayed in place to create more efficiency, by having two "supervisors" with specific responsibilities compared to one with overall charge, in the same department.

# Mutations are what created humans

Not all mutations are harmful. Some mutations of genes enable organisms—whether bacteria or humans—to live, thrive, adapt, and reproduce in unfavorable environments. The accumulation of gene mutations and the resulting new proteins they produce can change the specialization of cells, sizes, and the physical features of an organism for the better.

The ultimate evidence of beneficial genetic mutation is you—the present-day human being. Mutations affecting sperm or ovum have made our evolution possible. The best-studied evidence of mutations transmitted from our ancestors are the modifications seen in the size of our cranium to accommodate a larger brain, as well as changes in our muscles and bone structure that allowed us to walk upright. Another set of mutations led to changes in our teeth that enabled humans to bite and tear raw meat before fire was tamed and cooking became a common practice. Further mutations then changed our teeth to form a configuration that allows us to chew and break down cooked meat.

If we look backwards at our human evolution, we can see that the responses of our ancestors to their environment shaped the workings of the genes that we inherited and which we will pass to the next generations. They in turn will interact with an environment that will definitely be different from what our ancestors encountered. It is possible that in the future, other mutations will continue to create a further evolution of humans.

One critical thing to understand about gene mutations—they are irreversible. At this time, we have no evidence that mutations can be reversed, even if we change back to the prior environment in which we were living. In other words, mutations happening year after year have an additive effect because if they are codified at the cellular level, they are passed on to the next generation of cells.

## Not all adaptations lead to mutations

Darwin explained that changes that allow for greater survivability arise from conditions already present in the evolving organism.

However, not all adaptations that aid survivability need to be codified as mutations. One example is high altitude acclimatization. Nearly all oxygen carried by whole blood in humans is bound and transported by hemoglobin in red blood cells. When blood passes through the lungs, hemoglobin is about 96% saturated with oxygen. When passing through tissues almost 40% of oxygen is released. The release of oxygen is regulated by hemoglobin-associated molecules called *biphosphoglycerate* (BPG). The higher the BPG, the greater the release of oxygen.

If a healthy human is suddenly transported from sea level to about 8000 feet above sea level, the delivery of oxygen will be reduced because of lower oxygen levels in the air at higher altitudes. However, after a few hours at the higher altitude, BPG concentration begins to rise, causing release of more oxygen than normal. The situation is reversed when the person returns to sea level. This arrangement, supplemented by increased oxygen carrying capacity through the production of more red blood cells, allowed humans to survive at high altitudes for generations without experiencing mutation of the hemoglobin molecule.

Mutations that codified certain survival advantages sometimes produce collateral benefits in unexpected ways. For example, mutations for upright posture made it possible to walk on two legs for longer periods of time, and those for an opposable thumb made searching for food and escaping from physical threats easier. The vastly expanded visibility afforded when standing upright on two legs compared to crawling on four limbs, and a higher angle of vision to obtain a greater perception of our surroundings, must have forced the brain to not only enlarge in size but also make new nerve connections in profitable ways.

Combined, the human's increased awareness of self, the environment, and the interaction between the two created advances in art, literature, and science as we evolved. What's amazing is that, while the average difference in amino acid sequence in genes between humans and living African great apes is less than one percent, humans exhibit tremendous cultural capabilities simply due to better use of our central command center, the thinking brain.

# The causes of gene mutations

Mutations happen all the time due to many causes and most do not develop into cancer.

## Heredity

We all can inherit a mutated gene from a prior generation of our ancestors.

## Radiation

Ions (atoms stripped of electrons—such as from radioactive substances, gamma rays, X-rays, or ultraviolet light) have enough energy to break chemical bonds in a gene or cause the release of free radicals inside a cell that can damage the gene.

## Chemicals

Gene-damaging chemicals come from many sources, including naturally occurring components of plants and microbial organisms, fossil fuel before and after their combustion, synthetic products from industry, and even from some medical drugs. For example, benzene, hydroquinone, styrene, carbon tetrachloride, and trichloroethylene all have been recognized as gene-damaging chemicals.

The enzymes in charge of detoxification of chemicals that we consume can sometimes malfunction, making the chemical a potent cancer trigger. In addition, sometimes a chemical that has not been shown to cause gene mutation can do so under certain conditions. For example, the cancer-causing potential of some chemicals can be augmented by the presence of "promoters" such as hormones and drugs that help transmit signals in cells to manufacture materials or secrete growth-promoting factors. Exposure to a certain dosage of the chemical can change a cell's genes.

## Viruses

A virus can attach itself to the receptors on the cell and gain entry into the cell. Once inside, it is protected from immune system attack until it releases copies of itself to the outside. Some viruses can get incorporated into the genes causing mutations. However, viral infection does not automatically lead to gene malfunction even when it is integrated into the genetic material of the host, unless the location of the gene is a critical one.

## Free radicals

Metabolic activities inside a cell, exposure to radiation, and toxins can all lead to the production of "free radicals," which can damage cells. Normally, genes are located on the twisted ladder structure of two chromosome strands connected to each other by rungs of single hydrogen bonds. Usually hydrogen sits closer to one strand or the other. Free radicals can push the hydrogen molecule to the wrong side during the cell division, causing a gene mutation.

# What we know about mutations and their link to cancers

Evidence suggests that most cancers start in a single cell in which there are a sufficient number of mutations (probably a minimum of at least two mutations, such as in the growth-inhibiting genes).

Numerous findings demonstrate a link between certain mutations and specific cancers:

- Mutations of genes responsible for the production of growth-promoting factors have been implicated in brain, breast, bladder, and bone cancers.

- Mutations of genes responsible for producing signaling proteins have been implicated in colon, lung, pancreas, and skin cancers.

- Mutations of genes responsible for proteins that regulate the nuclear response to cell division signals have been implicated in cancer formation of lymphocytes, nerve cells, and in the lung.

These findings suggest that, just as an avalanche can start from any point on the side of a mountain, uncontrolled multiplication of cells can start due to mutation of genes at any point of the sequence that is responsible for cell proliferation.

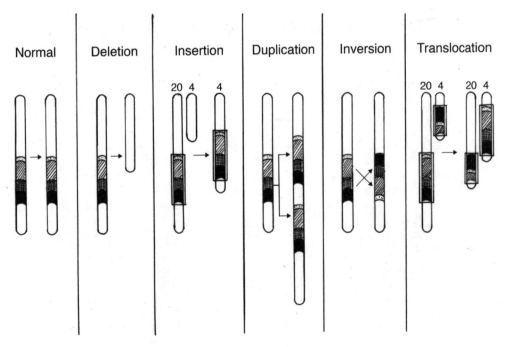

There are many types of possible mutations that can affect a gene. Each diagram here shows 1 gene and how the sequence of its DNA can be affected by a deletion, an extra insertion, a duplication, an inversion, or a translocation.

# It's the accumulation of mutations that counts

Cancer is not the result of mutation of a single gene inside a cell, but rather an accumulation of mutations in many genes over time, ultimately causing the cell to go haywire and begin a process of reproducing out of control. Cancer cells differ from normal cells in this regard. However, gene mutations do not automatically start cell multiplication and the initiation of cancer. But each cell multiplication has the potential to pass gene mutations forward, adding other mutations along the way. Let me explain.

During cell division, both strands of each chromosome in the nucleus duplicate from end to end. During the next hour, enzymes proofread these duplications, cut out defective areas and replace them with correct versions. However, any mistake that has already been incorporated into the genes from a prior generation will be reproduced as is, and passed on to the next generation of cells. Meanwhile, the potential for additional mutation increases with each event of cell multiplication, whatever the reason for multiplication may be.

Having two copies of every gene is usually our protection. For example, if there is a mutation in just one copy of the growth-activating gene and it starts a process of uncontrolled cell division, the growth-inhibiting gene should stop it. And even if there is a mutation in just one copy of the growth-inhibiting gene, the other should still function to halt the uncontrolled cell division. This double insurance offers some protection and is probably why cancer is not as widespread as it could be.

However, when there are mutations on both copies of the growth-inhibiting gene, there is no one to stop multiplication, thus uncontrolled cancerous cell division occurs.

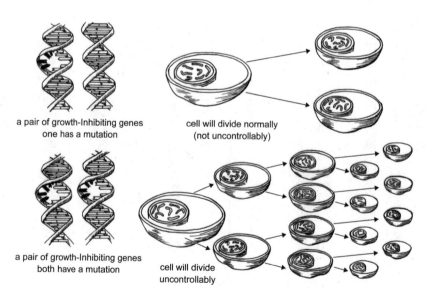

a pair of growth-Inhibiting genes
one has a mutation

cell will divide normally
(not uncontrollably)

a pair of growth-Inhibiting genes
both have a mutation

cell will divide
uncontrollably

A mutation on just one of the growth-inhibiting genes will still result in normal cell multiplication. But if both growth-inhibiting genes have a mutation, the cell will divide uncontrollably, leading to the potential for cancer.

# The science of some mutated genes

As mentioned earlier, cancer starts with a gene mutation urging the cell to divide uncontrollably as well as mutations of both growth-inhibiting genes (tumor suppressor genes).

Although cells with mutated genes may be able to multiply and develop into cancer, they still need to follow the guidelines established for multiplication of any normal cell in the body. This includes having a facilitating environment, the presence of signals to multiply, promoters that encourage cell division, and availability of nutrients needed for construction of new cells. They must also pass review from internal quality control inspectors and escape the scrutiny of external immune surveillance looking for abnormal multiplication activity.

Cancer cells, instead of having to circumvent each of these requirements, look for favorable environments and facilitator conditions that happen to occur in the body to start their clandestine activity. For example, cells in areas experiencing inflammation can release growth-promoting molecules into the local area. Cancer associated with chronic inflammatory bowel disease is an example of this.

Some mutated genes can act through intermediaries such as enzymes called *kinases* that outfit proteins with a phosphate module and make them "signaling" molecules. A mutant gene can produce hyperactive kinase workers that keep attaching phosphates to a number of proteins, completely changing the type or rate of activity inside a cell. Such a rogue kinase can keep on fitting proteins that are normally activated only during a cell division, leading to uncontrolled multiplication of the cell. Ordinarily, soon after the kinase enzyme completes the transfer of phosphate modules, another enzyme called *phosphatase* deactivates the active kinase. However, mutation of the gene responsible for the production of this phosphatase can lead to accelerated cell division.

# Inheriting gene mutations does not always lead to cancer

A history of cancer in families suggests that there may be a line of inherited defective genes passed from one generation to the next. But there are many individual factors relative to one's diet and environment that can affect your predisposition to cancer. For example, studies on identical twins who are raised by different parents in different environments show that if one twin develops cancer, it doesn't mean that the other twin will develop it in the same site.

However, the concordance for cancer is higher among monozygotic (identical) twins who share all genes than among dizygotic (fraternal) twins who, on average, share 50%. For example, the absolute risk of the same cancer before the age of 75 years for the monozygotic twin of a person with colorectal, breast, or prostate cancer was between 11 percent and 18 percent. By comparison, in dizygotic twins, who have the same degree of genetic similarity as full siblings, the risk of these cancers was 3 to 9 percent.[5]

Consider this analogy to understand the implications of your genetic inheritance. Your family is like a brand of cars that all have engines capable of speeds from zero to 120 mph. But each driver (every member of your family) determines the actual speed at which the car goes. In the same way, each of us is the driver of our genetic inheritance. Whether consciously or not, we influence the activation of those inherited genes through our dietary habits, exposure to toxins and environmental pollutants, and factors related to the strength of our immune system.

The conclusion among cancer specialists is that inherited genetic factors appear to contribute less than 20 percent to one's susceptibility to cancer, unless there is a specific inheritance pattern and detailed statistical analysis shows otherwise. This means that the increase in the risk of cancer even among close relatives is generally only moderate.

By contrast, genetic inheritance of some conditions other than cancer have a far higher risk of mortality. For example, the premature death of adults due to infections and vascular causes has a strong genetic background, and there is a fivefold increase in the mortality rate among adoptees living in different environments whose biologic parents died from infections.[6]

One reason that environment may be more influential than genetics is that although genes themselves contain recipes to make proteins, switches called *epigenetic tags* act upon a person's underlying genetic sequence to activate the genes. So even if you inherited genes identical to a twin who lived elsewhere, your epigenetic tags may not be activated due to a dissimilar environmental exposure. As a result, the expression of your inherited capabilities could be very different from that of your twin.

# Is cancer contagious?

In humans, cancer is not contagious. However, instances of cancer passing from one person to another are known, though extremely rare. For instance, the direct implantation of cancer cells from a laboratory or hospital environment and subsequent development of cancer has been noted in some humans. In another example, a melanoma cancer cell from a patient who was declared cured and later became a kidney donor was found thriving in the kidney recipient.

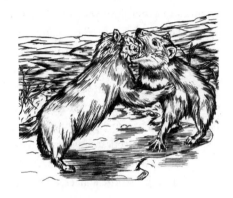

There is only one significant example of cancer being passed from one source to another. This is the "devil facial tumor disease" that affects Tasmanian Devils of Australia. When these animals fight, they often bite each other on the face. If cells from cancer on the face of one animal fall into the bite wound of another, the cancer cells survive in the recipient and start multiplying.

Ordinarily, when the immune system detects an intruder, such as bacteria or a mutated cell such as cancer, it is identified and destroyed. Why this does not occur in Tasmanian Devils is worth knowing.

It appears that cancer cells in the "devil facial tumor disease" do not activate the gene responsible for producing proteins that identify them. The reason for this is that these animals once lived in abundance on an island off the coast of Australia. When humans decided that they were a predatory nuisance, they were killed in large numbers. Later, when their population was found to be dropping rapidly, a breeding program was started to restore their numbers. Unfortunately, the stock available for the rebreeding program came from a very small surviving population. As a result of the inbreeding, most Tasmanian devils are closely related to each other and their cells do not recognize the invading cancer cells as foreign.

Sometimes the susceptibility to cancer can skip the person and appear in the next generation. The best example is a mother who takes *diethylstilbesterol* (DES) to prevent premature delivery. A daughter who is then exposed to the same chemical in utero may develop cancer later in her life. In 1971 the FDA advised US physicians not to use DES in pregnant women.

# So what caused MY cancer?

Everyone, even those who may suspect that they have an inherited tendency to develop cancer, will wonder, upon diagnosis, "What caused my cancer?" One motivation behind this question is to prevent a recurrence by knowing and thereby avoiding, if at all possible, the factors that caused it. In a world where one can access data related to the natural history of most infective agents and other illnesses, one expects to be able to know at least the circumstances, if not the specific agent, that caused the cancer.

However, no one can answer this question without knowing the natural growth history of the cancer. One would want to begin by assessing when it might have started. This is severely constrained by the limited availability of cancers for observation, study, and measurement. The questionable reliability of patients' recollections, the degree of acumen of the clinician, and the lack of ease in measurement of cancer can present further impediments. Even more detrimental for deciding the accurate history of a cancer is that by the time it is detected, it may have already completed a significant growth period.

Assuming that the cancer started as single cell, it would have had almost the same diameter of an ordinary cell, about $10\mu$ (microns). Assuming a volume of 1 cubic millimeter at the time of detection, 20 doublings would have been necessary for the original $10\mu$ diameter cell to gain that size. To reach the size needed for radiographic detection (1 centimeter in diameter), 10 additional cell divisions would have had to occur. This time between the cancer's inception and its detection, called the silent interval, usually takes up two-thirds of the tumor's total life span.

Can we work backwards, after measuring the size of a cancer, to calculate at least an approximate starting date? The simplest growth pattern would be one with regularly recurring cell division at fixed intervals, with one cell creating 2, 2 to 4, 4 to 8, and so on. However, for this to be reasonably accurate, one has to assume a constant tumor growth rate pattern over long periods of time, which is not necessarily the case for all cancers.

In short, it is often nearly impossible to look backwards to determine what precisely caused an individual's cancer or when it started.

# The mathematical calculation of tumor growth speed

Radiographic evaluation of measurable lung metastasis has shown a tumor-doubling time ranging from 11 to 164 days. A doubling time of less than 25 days is considered as rapid growth, 25 to 75 as intermediate, and slow if it exceeds 75 days.

So far, the most important information yielded by such evaluations is that clinical diagnosis is a late event in the natural history of cancer growth. For example, assuming a constant exponential growth, a very slow growing tumor with an initial detectability at the 1cm diameter may have had its inception between 10 and 25 years earlier. In other words, it is difficult even for a cancer specialist to help a patient get a feel for what may have started the cell to become cancerous.

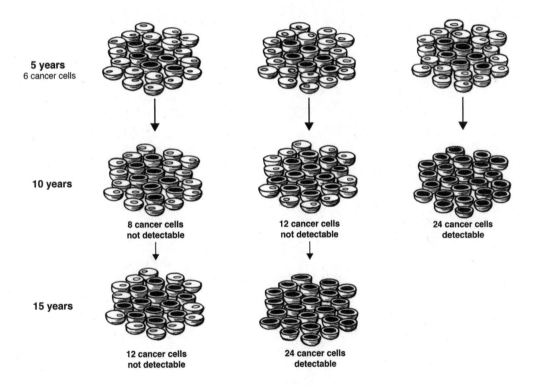

It is difficult to estimate when a cancer began. As this illustration shows, in the left column, 6 cancer cells multiplied very slowly and were not be detectable even after 15 years. The cancer in the middle column started with 6 cancer cells and grew such that it was not detectable after 10 years, but after 15 years was large enough to be detected. The cancer in the right column was fast growing and become detectable within 10 years. Many factors influence this growth rate.

# Some internal characteristics of cancer cells

THERE IS NO EVIDENCE TO SUGGEST THAT CANCER STARTS DUE TO A sudden weakness of the immune defense mechanism. The evolution of a cancer cell into a tumor requires activating multiple biological features that endow it with unique capabilities. In this section, I describe four capabilities that occur internally in a cancer cell that allow it to survive and multiply:

- being able to sustain the multiplication signal
- resisting apoptosis
- additional death-defying acts
- reprogramming energy production

Understanding these is the key to seeing the difficulty in treating cancer, as cancer treatment is currently practiced. This knowledge can also help you gain a new perspective on what I suggest you can do to survive cancer.

# How cancer cells sustain their multiplication

The division of a normal cell starts with signals from cells in its neighborhood, regardless of the location or type of cell involved. Receptors on the cell surface convey the message to the growth-activating gene, resulting in the production of a protein messenger to activate the duplication process. The multiplication then proceeds as a precise and coordinated event, with predictable activation of a sequence of genes.

A normal cell then stops division when the immediate need is met, whether this is healing a wound or forming a baby. Ordinarily, just contact with a neighboring cell is a strong enough signal to stop cell division.

As you can imagine, however, cancer cells manage to sustain multiplication. How do they do this?

Some cancer cells produce multiplication signal molecules themselves along with receptors that keep responding. Other cancer cells compel a compliant neighbor, usually a support cell, to generate signals and keep sending them. Still others may have mutations that can lead to the production of more signal receptors on the cell surface, making them hypersensitive. Some receptors may be mutated to the point of continuous internal signaling to multiply.

For example, almost 40% of human melanomas show mutated activity of the growth factor receptor. And other cancer cells benefit from a mutation that results in the failure of the normal mechanism that is supposed to stop the multiplication process. Development of certain types of leukemia is thought to be due to no responsiveness to proliferation suppressors.

While most cells suppress further proliferation when they come in contact with their neighbor, cancer cells continue the process.

# The mechanism of sustained multiplication signaling in cancer cells

Cells are programmed to respond to signals for multiplication transmitted from one cell to its neighbor proportional to the number and position of cells needed in a particular organ or tissue to maintain normal structure and function. Once the messenger molecule binds to a receptor on the cell membrane, it sends signals via branched intracellular signaling pathways notifying machinery inside the cell to awaken the genes in charge of cell division inside the nucleus.

In some cancer cells, the nucleus may have a defective gene sending out instructions to keep the multiplication process going. This is similar to relay stations transmitting signals around the earth through a number of different satellites. If one instrument is stuck in transmission mode, copy after copy of the message may be forwarded from the malfunctioning equipment. The receiving stations, having no way of knowing the situation, will keep sending them onwards. In the same way, mutations may disarm a cell's normal responsiveness to signals from neighboring cells to stop the process of multiplication.

In some cancers, uncontrolled multiplication signals occur only when there is a trigger. However, it can take months or even years for a trigger. It took five years after the nuclear attacks on Hiroshima and Nagasaki for the appearance of leukemia among those who were exposed to radiation.

The trigger could be the presence of growth promoters such as hormones. These can accelerate the multiplication of cancer cells. Estrogen is one such hormone. According to the results of a study released by the National Cancer Institute, women who take birth control pills tend to have higher cancer risk compared to the women who don't. Long-term use of any type of female hormones to ease menopause symptoms also raises the risk of breast cancer in women. Similarly, the intake of growth hormone may be a risk factor for cancer development.

# How normal cells stop multiplication and self-destruct

Every cell in the body contains a pair of growth-inhibiting genes that are supposed to play a vital role in stopping a cancer cell from multiplying.[7] They are in charge of interpreting signals from neighboring cells that provide warnings about indiscriminate growth and encroachment on them. If this message is received, the growth-inhibiting gene is supposed to initiate steps to halt the cell division or to have the cell self-destruct, which we discussed earlier as the process called *apoptosis*.

Apoptosis is a genetically regulated process that is essential for the proper development of the size and shape of organs. On the other hand, cells that are supposed to last a lifetime, such as nerve cells, must resist a signal for apoptosis, even if it results in improper nerve function.

A mutation of one copy of the growth-inhibiting gene will not affect this function, since the other copy can take over the job. However, when there is a mutation in both growth-inhibiting genes, the person is out of luck—the body has no mechanism to halt the multiplication of cancer cells with these mutated genes.

A mutation in both genes at a young age predisposes a person to childhood cancer, or to an increased lifetime risk of cancer and the potential for multiple tumors. In an adult, a mutation on both copies of the growth-inhibiting gene is likely to contribute to the uncontrolled multiplication of cancer cells.

In many cancers, both growth-activating and growth-inhibiting genes have mutated, resulting in the production of a cell line that could become highly cancerous. On the other side are people with Down syndrome in whom solid cancers are believed to be less common due to increased expression of growth-inhibiting genes.

**CURIOUS TIDBITS**

It turns out that elephants have multiple copies of growth-inhibiting genes. This likely explains why they have a low incidence of cancer, as it appears that they can more efficiently stop cells with mutated genes from multiplying rather than trying to repair the genes without success, as happens in humans. This could be nature's way of protecting an animal with a high rate of cell division and the periodic availability of hormones (in female elephants) that promote growth but also set the stage for cancer to occur.

# The mechanism of how cancer cells resist apoptosis

Programmed cell death serves as a natural prevention of cancer formation. Genes in charge of self-destruction activate the process if they detect an abnormality in the intracellular operating system, or sense overwhelming or irreparable damage to cellular subsystems.

A protein called *cytochrome c,* usually held inside the mitochondria, is released in response to the apoptosis signal. Once outside, it activates enzymes to carry out the apoptosis.

The apoptosis machinery has two components. One responds to growth-inhibitory signals that originate largely outside of the cell, and the other is in charge of intracellular operating systems.

Once the growth-inhibiting gene verifies abnormal activity of genes in charge of cell multiplication, it initiates the steps necessary to correct it, first by identifying the source. It might be a gene stuck in the transmission mode, a relay station continuing to send messengers to keep the process going, or one station not responding to signals to stop the activity. If the attempt to stop the process of cell division is not successful, the gene will initiate the second component, a self-destruction sequence that results in cell death. Ordinarily, regulatory proteins bound to the apoptosis trigger gene prevent its activation, but now the apoptosis machinery springs into action, resulting in cell death.

Cancer cells show a variety of strategies to circumvent apoptosis. One is the modification of gene activity related to signals of critical intracellular events. Another way is by under-producing agents that act as sensors of critical activities. A third is by reducing the number of agents needed to start the self-destruction process.

## CURIOUS TIDBITS

- It has been shown that *aflatoxin*, a product of a fungus that contaminates improperly stored commodities such as cassava, chili peppers, corn, cotton seed, millet, peanuts, rice, sorghum, sunflower seeds, tree nuts, wheat, and a variety of spices can interfere with the work of growth-inhibiting genes, leading to liver cancer.[8]

- Non-organic particulate matter such as asbestos can not only produce chronic inflammation and accelerated cell reproduction, but can also, because its particles are so small, get into a cell and interfere with the function of the growth-inhibiting gene. The result is continued cell multiplication and cancer formation.

- The human papilloma virus (HPV) causes cancer by deactivating the growth-inhibiting gene, allowing those cells to multiply out of control. Out of over 170 HPV types, about a dozen are linked to cancer of the cervix, eight to that of the lungs and two to an increasing number of head and neck cancers. In fact, these HPV-caused head and neck cancers will outnumber (in the US) cervical cancer in the next decade or two.

# Additional death-defying acts in cancer cells

There are three additional actions that cancer cells can take to survive.

1.  Most cell lines in the body are able to pass through only a limited number of successive cell growth-and-division cycles. This has to do with *telomeres*, which are protective caps on chromosomes that are supposed to prevent them from fusing with each other. Each time a normal cell divides, the telomeres are shortened. With each cell division, the genes become shorter and shorter, and eventually the cell loses its ability to multiply. Some cancer cells incapacitate the gene that controls the telomere removal, and thus the cells keep multiplying.

2.  However, in cells that are designed to divide extensively, such as in stem cells, there is an enzyme called *telomerase*, programmed to add length to telomeres so that the genes maintain their capacity to multiply. Here too, cancer cells can wreak havoc, by activating this enzyme and causing cells to continue multiplying. Telomerase activation has been observed in 90% of all human tumors.[9]

3.  Autophagy is a mechanism available to normal cells experiencing extreme nutrient deficiency that enables them to survive until nutrient availability is restored. During this process, cells break down their internal cellular organelles, including mitochondria, and use the dismantled parts for structural support, while energy production and use are maintained at just a survival level. Then when nutrient availability is restored, the cell can manufacture the dismantled parts back to functional capability. However, some cancer cells, upon receiving the instruction to self-destruct, use this same physiological mechanism to survive until the environment is conducive for their growth.

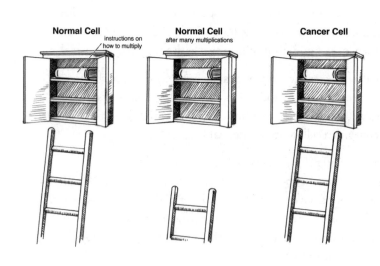

**Normal Cell**
instructions on how to multiply

**Normal Cell**
after many multiplications

**Cancer Cell**

Telomeres are the caps at the ends of chromosomes. Each time a cell divides, a piece of the telomere disappears, similar to a ladder getting shorter and shorter with use, so that after many cell divisions, the cell can no longer divide. However, cancer cells can deactivate the telomere shortening process, which allows them to keep multiplying.

# More on cancer cell mechanisms to resist self-destruction

One of the natural mechanisms used by the body to eliminate a non-functioning or unwanted cell is by the creation of a radical called reactive oxygen species (ROS) whose toxicity can lead to cell death. But to moderate the damaging consequences of ROS, normal cells also produce a neutralizing protein. A number of human cancers produce an excess of the protein designed to neutralize ROS and escape apoptosis.[10]

Cancer cells have several additional mechanisms to resist self-destruction. One of these explains the link between smoking and cancer. Tobacco smoke contains *benzopyrene*, which can cause a mutation in the gene responsible for programmed cell death by interfering with "telomere shortening," allowing cells to continue multiplication and become cancerous.

Hibernation with or without autophagy is another way cancer cells can achieve self-preservation. After receiving the signal to self-destruct, a cancer cell can initiate activities to circumvent its execution first by incapacitating the mitochondrion. This immediately reduces the energy supply to the control mechanisms, such that they cannot send out distress signals or alert the immune system. Without a functioning mitochondrion, the cytochrome c also cannot move out to start the activation of the workers in charge of dismantling cell structure.

In addition, a cancer cell can suspend almost all activities that can be detected as evidence of life by external sensors and go into hibernation. This allows it to maintain the potential to become active at a later stage when the conditions are just right. There is incontestable evidence in the literature detailing remarkably long—three decades or more—silent periods between rapid proliferations of cancer cells.[11]

This is yet another reason why the phrase "five-year cure" is not appropriate when it comes to cancer treatment.

# Cancer cells can reprogram their production of energy

As you learned, cells are driven to survive because they are programmed from the Adam Cell to multiply. Once the instruction for multiplication has been received, the cell machinery swings into action. Its two most urgent actions are: securing a reliable and continuous source for energy production, and securing all needed raw materials.

In general, normal cells use the power generation facility called the mitochondrion to extract maximum energy from the nutrients we consume. Recall that the mitochondria can convert either glucose or fatty acids to create ATP, the fuel that powers the cell's metabolic processes.

Cancer cells behave differently; they are almost cunning. When a cancer cell divides, it has little interest in creating the usual structures of the cells from which it originated. Perhaps because the mutation has incapacitated it, it is driven only to survive, needing only the barest amount of functionality. Other than routine maintenance, the cancer cell has no intention or need to perform as part of the tissue it was assigned to. This is not unlike how the cell behaved in its Adam Cell mode, when function and collaboration with other cells had no role in its life.

As a result, the main goal of the cancer cell is to gain enough energy to multiply. One thing cancer cells do is incapacitate the mitochondria. Even without functioning mitochondria, the cell can continue the less efficient process of breaking down glucose outside the mitochondria. Although this is a more primitive method of getting energy, it at least provides enough energy for the cancer cell to multiply. In addition, glycolysis itself leads to the production of raw materials that can be used to construct structures for new cells.

The upshot of this is that cancer cells *crave* glucose. To ensure a steady supply of fuel for energy production, cancer cells begin creating multiple types of "glucose transporters" that literally suck glucose from the outside into the cell to make ATP. This allows cancer cells to not be dependent on the presence of insulin outside the cell to promote glucose uptake through the cell wall.

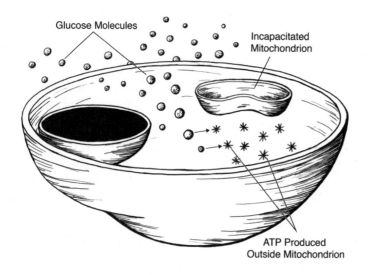

Glucose Molecules

Incapacitated Mitochondrion

ATP Produced Outside Mitochondrion

Normal cells can use glucose or fatty acids inside their mitochondria to make ATP. Because cancer cells incapacitate their mitochondria, they must rely solely on glucose to produce ATP energy outside the mitochondria. The upshot of this is that cancer cells crave glucose.

# Why cancer alters the energy production within a cell

Mitochondria can produce ATP molecules from Acetyl Co-A, a product derived from fatty acid, amino acid, or glucose because one metabolite called *oxaloacetate* from glucose utilization can be reutilized. In type 1 diabetics, lack of insulin prevents entry of needed glucose into muscle cells to produce energy from glycolysis alone. In addition, some of the oxaloacetate produced is drawn off to the liver to produce glucose that neurons in the brain prefer as fuel, resulting in the accumulation of small fatty acids compounds, precursors of Acetyl Co-A, also known as ketone bodies, creating diabetic ketoacidosis.

In contrast, a cancer cell can survive without needing power from mitochondria.[12] Why does a cancer cell intentionally not use energy generated by mitochondria?

1. The lower power generation capacity helps mask the cancer cell's non-participation in functional performance, thereby avoiding the internal scrutiny of a mismatch between energy production and metabolic activity of the cell.

2. It allows the cancer cell to utilize nutrients that would have been used for other metabolic activities the cell was expected to perform, to fabricate new cancer cells instead.

3. Cells are programmed to initiate apoptosis when mitochondria become incapable of producing ATP. A cancer cell can evade this process by not activating mitochondria in the first place.

4. Yet another reason is a forward-looking one. Materials such as lactate released from incomplete degradation of glucose lead to changes in the neighborhood and aid in the migration of cancer cells, as you will learn later.

Thus, blocking or not activating genes responsible for the normal functionality of the cell, including monitoring of the power generation capability inside mitochondria, may be an important evasive methodology for cancer cells to survive and spread.

## CURIOUS TIDBITS

In a small percentage of thyroid cancers (15%), the cancer cells find a way to continue their clandestine activity while continuing the production of thyroid hormone, an activity they were expected to perform. To do this, they need a reliable energy supply. They accomplish this by generating energy in functional mitochondria. In other words, these tumors may have two subpopulations of cancer cells that differ in their energy generating capabilities. While the regular cancer cells extract ATP from glucose and release lactate to the outside as waste, cells in the second subpopulation take in lactate to functioning mitochondria and extract ATP, utilizing oxygen. This, it may be surprising to learn, is not an invention of cancer cells but an expression of a normal physiological ability such as seen in muscle fibers producing energy under less than optimal oxygen conditions.

# Some external characteristics of thriving cancer cells

IN THIS SECTION, I DESCRIBE FOUR CAPABILITIES MANIFESTED BY cancer that help them multiply and thrive:

- inducing blood vessel formation
- evading immune surveillance
- sending scouts to select sites for settlement - metastasis
- utilizing local cells and their environment for metastasis

# How cancer cells induce blood vessel formation

Cancer cells require nutrients and oxygen for cellular functions as well as an outlet to remove waste and carbon dioxide. To accomplish these things, cancer cells release messengers to go outside the cell with instructions to construct new blood vessels and connect them to any available blood vessels in the vicinity. This ensures a steady supply of needed materials for construction of new cancer cells.

Both the Phase 1 embryonic cells and Phase 2 tissue specific stem cells are able to activate the gene that facilitates the growth of blood vessels. Embryonic cells have the capability to produce cells that can be fashioned into tubes connecting to each other to form entire circulatory conduits. In addition, they produce signaling agents to induce sprouting of new blood vessels from existing ones.

This capability is actually normal and can be activated under two circumstances. One is for wound healing and the other occurs during the female menstrual cycle. But while these are temporary in normal cell activity, during cancer progression the triggers for new blood vessel formation remain active to induce an almost continuous sprouting of new vessels that help sustain the ability of cancer cells to acquire the nutrients they need.

This activation of new blood vessel formation happens very early during the development of cancer. It is continuously sustained, but the blood vessels produced are not uniform like a normally fashioned vessel. They are convoluted at times, distorted with excessive branching and irregular internal diameters. This leads to them being erratic in sustaining circulation and subject to leakiness. However, the strategy seems to serve a useful purpose—keeping cancer cells alive and thriving.

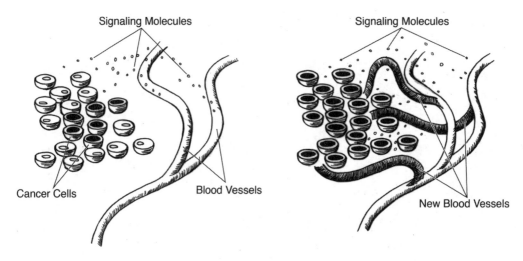

Cancer cells can send out signaling molecules to tell nearby blood vessels to generate new branches to supply the cancer cells with more nutrients.

# The mechanism of new blood vessel formation

There is a signaling protein in normal cells called *vascular endothelial growth factor-A* that is released during embryonic development. This protein binds to receptors on the surface of an existing blood vessel to orchestrate new vessel growth. After a blockage of an artery supplying blood to the heart muscle, new blood vessels are formed to bypass the obstructed area to supply oxygen and nutrients to help the tissue survive and repair. This is an example of functionally useful new blood vessel formation between adjacent blood vessels.

Cancer cells are known to release the signaling protein as a mechanism to promote new blood vessel growth. In addition, they can induce neighboring cells to release agents that sustain new blood vessel formation. Although such activation of new blood vessel formation occurs early in the life of a cancer, the progression of new blood vessel formation is erratic.

Another mechanism that helps the formation of new blood vessels is the arrival of immune cells capable of releasing signals for construction to make it easier for establishing supply lines. Infections that attract immune cells thus can assist cancer cell growth.

The body has natural inhibitors that aim to prevent unneeded vessel formation, such as when a wound has healed. But cancer cells can disable these inhibitors to keep the process going.

# Cancer cells can evade immune surveillance

One might expect the normal immune system to eradicate the formation of a new cancer, or resist the aggressive progression of an established cancer, or prohibit a cancer from setting up satellite colonies in another part of the body. Yet, cancers often develop in people who appear to have normal defense mechanisms, effective against other diseases.

The reason is that cunning cancer cells often develop ways to evade the surveillance of the immune system cells. Their ruse is perpetrated in several ways.

First, cancer cells may eliminate or reduce the expression of "identification proteins" on their cell membranes that would normally attract the attention of the immune system. Some cancer cells shed proteins that would normally attract Natural Killer cells in the vicinity, to mislead them. This allows them to continue their multiplication process, while the killers are following the wrong signals. For example, prostate cancer cells can release a large amount of proteins into the bloodstream that immune cells can chase, while they continue living undisturbed. This is similar to counter-intelligence agents removing the shoe embedded with a signal-producing device from an operative and sending it in a different direction to mislead the tracking ability of the spies. Prostate cancer is notorious for this type of evasion.

In addition, some cancers surround and incorporate healthy cells that continue to produce and release proteins normal for that tissue. This, of course, fools the immune system into perceiving the cancer as functioning normally. Some thyroid cancers do this.

Some cancers not only subvert the intent of immune cells, but also recruit them as sentinels to protect themselves. The compromised immune cells make cancer cells less responsive to radiation and chemotherapy. In addition, as mentioned earlier, the compromised immune cells may be further programmed into releasing molecules that promote the growth of tiny blood vessels that bring even more glucose and other nutrients to the vicinity of cancer cells.

Even if the immune system has been alerted, what appears to happen in some people is that the cancer cell multiplication occurs very fast, outpacing the arrival of adequate immune cells to destroy them. This is similar to the worsening of a simple infection while your immune system is cranking up to mount an attack against the invaders. The pace of the infection is simply too quick for the immune response.

# The mechanism of evading immune destruction

There is no question that the incidence of certain cancers is high in people with defective immune systems. However, viruses cause most of these cancers when the viral load overwhelms the immune system. Yet, although more and more cancers are found to be viral related, the majority of tumors are not in people with compromised immune systems. So, what exactly is the role of the immune system in halting cancer?

Studies using genetically engineered mice showed that deficiencies in the development or function of specific immune cells do indeed contribute to an increased incidence of cancers of both viral and non-viral origin. For example, in one study, cancer cells transplanted from immunodeficient mice did not survive in immunocompetent mice, whereas cancer cells from immunocompetent mice were efficient at establishing themselves in both competent and deficient mice populations. [13,14]

This means that a competent immune system should be able to eliminate cancers that can be identified. For example, it has been established that patients with colon and ovarian cancers that are heavily infiltrated with immune cells have a better prognosis than those with less infiltration of killer (immune) cells.

However, recall that cancer cells have many ways to mask their true identity. Some cancer cells secrete agents that directly suppress immune cells, while others recruit cells that mediate inflammation as active participants to incapacitate immune cells. Such ruses help them grow without interference from immune cells. Some organ transplant recipients who take immuno-suppressing agents develop cancer, which has been shown to be transplanted into their body as part of the organ from a person perceived to be tumor free after successful treatment. Keep in mind that immunosuppression used as part of transplant therapy could facilitate the development of a cancer in the recipient.

# Metastasis: How cancer cells multiply

A cancer cell appears at random and most will remain solitary at the site of origin. However, some can multiply and spread. The most feared characteristic of cancer is its colonization of other parts of the body. When this happens, it is called *metastasis*.

A solitary cancer can cause different symptoms depending on where it is located. It can obstruct the flow of air in bronchial tubes, impede fluid flow in the urinary tract, block the passage of solid waste in the bowel, or stop secretions in whatever organ it inhabits. For the most part, if cancer stays in the immediate area of initial appearance, such as a localized tumor, it results in non-fatal consequences, as the tumor can be removed.

When a cell detaches itself from the group and starts its solo journey, it is exhibiting one of the fundamental properties that distinguish a life form from everything else that exists in the universe. Only a living cell can move from one location to another, on its own. Normal cells can also get detached from their home location (the tissue or organ where they began life). But when this happens, they will usually initiate a programmed cell death routine. For cancer cells, however, they are reclaiming, thanks to their genetic mutations, their original ability to act and live independently outside of the organ or tissue of which they are supposed to be a partner.

Cancer cells that detach may also self-destruct, but some may manage to live on and migrate to start a colony almost anywhere in the body, in an unpredictable way. Even though we expect regional lymph nodes to block the travel of cancer cells through the lymphatic channels, some manage to squeeze through to continue their journey to a location far from where they originated.

Once the process of migration starts, millions of cancer cells can be released to wander about in all parts of the body. Just as humans do during migration from one land area to another, cancer cells may also start as small groups, then divide to even smaller groups to overcome the difficulties encountered during the journey so that at least some reach destinations previously unknown to them.

Many cancer cells may start the journey, only to be stopped and destroyed by surveillance mechanisms or lack of nutrients, similar to the fate of human explorers of the past and future. However, unlike humans, survival of even one cancer cell is enough to launch a new colony, multiplying and multiplying many times over.

# The mechanisms of cancer cell scouting

Every cell in a tissue or organ is attached to at least some of its neighbors by protein molecules similar to how two papers can be glued together. So the first step in cancer cell migration is altering the cell-to-cell adhesion molecules. Although simple degradation may be enough to detach from the neighbor, some cancer cells replace the adhesion molecule with one that was present during its embryonic state so that when it reaches a distant site it is more likely to be accepted by its new neighbors.

After detachment, the cell starts the journey by penetrating blood vessels, lymph vessels, or body cavities. The most successful methodology for spreading and escaping the surveillance mechanisms that are trained to ignore embryonic cells is to transform into the earlier phase of a cell—the stem cell phase. This allows cancer cells to burrow into neighboring tissues, similar to what an embryo does in the placenta. In addition, they take materials from destroyed cells for their own use.

Unlike normal cells, cancer cells produce lactate as the end product of glycolysis. The lactate released to the outside changes the extracellular acidity. Ordinarily, the body strictly maintains local acidity by allowing a variation of only about one millionth compared with variations in ions such as sodium. While ordinary cells cannot tolerate an acidic environment and recede, cancer cells thrive, thus increasing the size of cancer proportional to lactate levels.[15]

To drain the acidic material, the body activates enzymes that digest tissue. Cancer cells move through the newly formed channels to the nearest blood vessel, release enzymes to digest vessel walls, gain entry into the bloodstream, and ride to other parts of the body. Attempts by the body to repair the leaky vessel could also be hijacked by signaling molecules that cancer cells release to start the construction of new blood vessels for their own convenience.

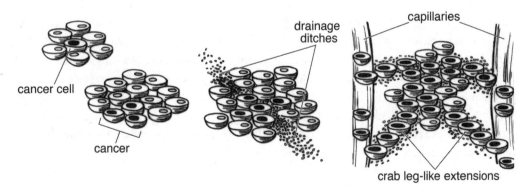

Cancer cells produce lactate as a result of glucose utilization for energy production. Normal cells cannot tolerate the acidic environment caused by lactate and recede from the area of the cancer cell. In addition, the presence of lactate activates local enzymes capable of digesting the protective matrix around cells, so as to drain the acidic material. Cancer cells take advantage of the drainage channels to move through them to the nearest blood vessel. This process makes cancer growth take on a crab-like shape. Cancer was thus named after the Greek zodiac sign Cancer, for the crab.

# How cancer cells utilize local cells and their environment for metastasis

There is general consensus among medical doctors that the major cause of cancer-related morbidity and mortality is when a cancer metastasizes and establishes colonies away from its site of origin.* If a cancer metastasizes to other sites, it dramatically increases the likelihood of death. In fact, it has been estimated that the main cause of death in 90% of patients diagnosed with a solid tumor is the migration, invasiveness, and secondary growth of cancer in distant sites. Most cancers have the ability to metastasize. Only one of the most common cancers in the United States, basal cell cancer of the skin, has an extremely low metastatic rate.

A solitary cancer can be misleading. A newly detected tumor in the lungs, for example, may appear to be solitary. But if the cell structure does not match that of the lung tissue, it could have originated in another part of the body such as the breast and got stuck in the lungs while travelling through the circulation. The finding that cancer cells are made of abnormal breast cells, not abnormal lung cells, reveals its true nature. As such, it will be called metastatic breast cancer, not lung cancer.

The process of how cancer cells find a neighborhood, often having no resemblance to where they came from, while evading the scrutiny of their new neighbors is still not clearly understood.

For example, cancer cells from one breast rarely go to the other breast to start a new colony even though the environment in the breast tissue is more similar to the one from where their journey started. Rather they tend to go elsewhere, such as to the lungs. Similarly, cancer cells from the prostate gland can find accommodating neighbors in the lung without much difficulty. In fact, adaptation to local conditions and activation of genes to facilitate survival in an unfamiliar environment seem to happen faster than previously thought.

As they grow, cancer cells invade their neighbors without respecting normal boundaries. Multiplying in a confined area such as the bone marrow crowds out other cells that originally occupied that space, creating a reduced number of functional cells to maintain needed services at the level required for the survival of the body. This can lead to complications such as anemia due to diminished production of red blood cells, inability to fight infections due to reduced production of immune cells, and increased tendency to bleed due to inadequate production of platelets needed to form clots in a timely manner to plug a hole in a blood vessel. Cancer cells spreading out in a confined space such as the skull may compress other cells in the brain, creating functional difficulties depending on the areas compressed, headaches, nausea due to increased intracranial pressure, and even seizures.

---

* Bronchioloalveolar carcinoma (BAC) of the lung is a rare exception. It is the only cancer, though localized, that can kill directly. Imagine cancer cells growing in a culture dish in the laboratory. The cells will keep multiplying on the surface of culture exposed to air on the outside and in contact with nutrients underneath. Depending on the virulence of growth, cancer cells can spread covering the medium completely, similar to oil spreading on water, and even going over sides of the dish. In other words, cancer cells can prevent contact between the culture medium and air. Similarly, cancer cells of BAC can spread over the surface of the lung air sacs interfering with the transfer of oxygen molecules into the blood, resulting in gradual suffocation and death.

# The mechanism of metastatic colonization

Most cancer cells grow more rapidly than the rate of growth of cells of the tissue they are part of, but their growth may not be constant over time. Instead, they may enter a period of dormancy lasting for years. In rare cases, the growth may stop and the cells even disappear spontaneously. On the other hand, there may be a period of dormancy followed by a sudden spurt of growth. Insufficient availability of needed nutrients for energy generation, anti-growth signals from local cells, or tumor-suppressing actions of immune cells can all impede vigorous colony growth.

In some cases, however, a growth spurt of small metastatic cells starts immediately after removal of a cancer tumor, indicating that perhaps molecules released for new blood vessel formation required for healing the surgical wound found their way to the dormant cancer cells.

Most cancer cells are foreign to the environment outside the new colony and may need time to become adapted to the neighborhood and neighbors. However, certain tissue environments, especially the liver and lungs, turn out to be very hospitable compared to others. This could be because these organs often experience a high rate of inflammation or injury from ingested and inhaled noxious agents. This causes them to release signaling molecules asking for help for fighting or healing. Meanwhile, freely floating cancer cells simply follow the signaling markers to the site of these organs, where they are welcomed as "helpers" responding to the need.

Once in place, they appear friendly to the local immune cells. They even release signaling molecules of their own to promote the formation of new blood vessels, which immune cells interpret as helping the flow of materials needed to meet the local need. Many cancer cells produce protein markers normally present only on fetal cells, allowing them to escape surveillance by immune cells.

By the time the immune system detects that the cells are actually cancer, they may have grown to have such strength in numbers that it overwhelms the local immune system.

Two other sites—bones and the brain—are also highly prone to metastases. Because they usually experience very little exposure to noxious agents, they do not have a vigilant local immune system to detect cancer cells that happen to get stranded in them. When that happens, the cancer can spread before the immune system has a chance to stop it.

# Some cancer-enabling factors of the body

In this section, I describe four facilitative factors that help cancer cells activate their characteristics and enable cancer to behave in its unique ways:

- gene mutations
- the role of inflammation
- chronic cell regeneration
- elevated blood glucose level

# Factors causing gene mutations

First, you should remember that genes mutate all the time, but not every mutation holds. As you recall, adaptations allow cells to survive under the stress of an adverse environment. The adapted cell can pass on its new capability to daughter cells so that they may survive the same challenge. However, the challenge faced by the daughter cells may not be the same as that of the parent cell. This means that there is no advantage in codifying adaptive capability through a gene mutation to be passed on to the next generation, unless that particular challenge persists over time.

So when a mutation happens, what are the factors that might cause it to stick? Are mutations more influenced by exposure to cancer-causing agents, or is one's age more important?

The incidence rate of a cancer at a particular age is the proportion per unit of time of people of that age who develop a particular cancer. The strongest determinant of gene mutations resulting in cancer incidence rates appears to be age. For example, the probability that a man will develop cancer in the next five years is 1 in 14 if he is 65, but only 1 in 700 if he is 25. This relative risk is 50 to 1. Differences in cancer incidence rates between young adults and old adults of this order of magnitude are found in many species other than humans.

The question is whether these marked increases with age arise because of exposure to cancer-causing agents causing mutations that accumulate over time—or whether they arise because aging decreases the capability of our immune system to perform effective surveillance of cancer cells, or both? This question may have been answered by an experiment involving 950 mice with a normal lifespan of 2-3 years. In laboratory conditions, the same cancer-causing agent was applied to the skin starting at 10, 25, 40, or 55 weeks of age. The incidence rate of cancer among the mice in each group increased steeply with time. However, the increase was independent of the age at which the mice received exposure. Rather, the incidence was proportional with the duration of time the mice were exposed. For example, mice of any age exposed for longer durations had a higher incidence of cancer than mice that received less exposure.[16]

This means that lifelong regular exposure of humans to mutation-causing agents such as cigarette smoke will be more dangerous the younger one's exposure starts. Escape of even one mutated cell from immune destruction is enough for the cell to sustain more mutations and pass on the accumulated mutations to daughter cells. In short, as time passes, gene mutations due to mistakes during cell divisions accumulate proportional to the rate of cell divisions.

# The challenge of detecting mutations

German physician Paul Ehrlich (1854-1915) proposed in 1909 that mutated cells arise continuously and that the immune system eradicates these before they become established in the body. He also pioneered the cultivation of tumor cells by transplanting them to test their virulence and survival skills. In the mid-20th century, tumor transplantation studies suggested the existence of telltale proteins associated with mutated cells that could be identified by our immune surveillance mechanisms.

The human immune system is designed to distinguish "self" from "non-self" and then destroy what is identified as non-self, such as viruses, bacteria or other pathogens that may be a threat to the body. The binding of suspicious proteins to receptors on the surface of white blood cells is usually the first step in initiating an immune response, which is a very intricate process coordinated between many classes of molecules and cell types.

Ordinarily, when neighborhood cells detect an abnormal growth, they will release messenger proteins to the offending cell. If the offending cell continues its multiplication, the neighboring cells alert the immune system. The immune system will then try to induce the self-destruction of the offending cell. If that does not work, it can bring in reinforcements such as killer cells to destroy the offending cell.

However, the immune system may be unable to identify a cell multiplying uncontrollably, as it can appear normal from the outside. In addition, mutated genes hide behind two protective walls: a nuclear membrane and a cell membrane. The last thing immune cells want to do is to destroy normal cells. On some occasions, cancer cells, aware of the intense immune activity in the neighborhood, may even decide to forego further multiplication for the time being. The result could a solitary cancer that one may die with, rather than die from.

## CURIOUS TIDBITS

Human immunodeficiency virus, the virus that causes AIDS (acquired immune deficiency syndrome) infects the white cells in charge of detecting the proteins released by them. This strategy progressively incapacitates the entire immune system.

# The role of inflammation in helping cancer cells

It has been estimated that about 15 percent of cancers worldwide can be attributed to infections.[17] Recent data suggest that inflammation, a natural process of infection control and wound healing, is an ideal set up for formation of cancer cells.[18] For example, chronic inflammation, and the associated repeated cycles of cell death and regeneration, favor the occurrence of gene mutations. Continued presence of an infectious agent, due to the inability of the immune system to eliminate it, can be responsible for chronic inflammation. Or an inert material such as asbestos fibers that local enzymes find difficult to digest can cause damage to normal tissues and the development of chronic inflammation. In addition to repeated cell regeneration, infectious agents can also directly change genes and compromise the immune cells—thus facilitating cancer formation.

Normally, inflammation is a sign of frenzied biochemical and cellular activity. The purpose of inflammation is to destroy a foreign agent that is perceived to cause cell injury, or at least to wall off the area of inflammation from the surrounding normal cells and repair the damaged tissue. Rehabilitating the cells back to normalcy, and/or filling the defect with fibroblasts that form scar tissue is how repair is done.

It is during the repair process that cancer can invade. Here's how. The repair process starts with a number of signaling molecules released by injured cells. These signaling molecules attract circulating immune cells to the site, and neighboring resident cells render aid. However, the activity of immune cells to destroy the infective agent releases free radicals. This can damage genes in a newly forming cell as well as a resident cell. The vast majority of cells with damaged genes will be instructed to self-destruct and will then be removed.

The main problem, however, is that signals released during inflammation may attract travelling cancer cells to the location where they can be welcomed by resident cells and ignored by immune cells—the right conditions for metastasis to occur.

Cells in the area of the infection, normally vigilant about intruders, are forced to tolerate and even help in the production of new cells in the neighborhood. They may not only let their guard down but may even assist with the establishment of cancer cells that ordinarily would not have been allowed to stay, without being aware of their true nature. It may be too late by the time cells outside the immediate area recognize the truth.

# Inflammation: A welcome mat for cancer cell entry and residence

One of the locations cancer cells often successfully develop and/or embed themselves in is a site of inflammation. A basic understanding of the workings of inflammation will help you to learn about how cancer spreads this way.

Inflammation starts when specialized cells that carry protein samples from the infective agent go to the regional lymph node where specific antibodies that can identify and even attack the infective agent are manufactured. Immune cells armed with a specific seek-and-destroy function to eradicate the infective agent are then sent out.

What happens when they arrive is as follows. Just like a car accident on a road causes traffic to slow down, in the same way, when there is injury to a body part, circulation through tiny blood vessels called capillaries slows down so that immune cells that would have ordinarily passed through can come into contact with adhesive materials laid down by the lining of the capillary to mark the site of injury. Immune cells can now get out through openings in the capillary wall and move in the direction of the signaling agents released by injured cells or proteins coming from the infective agent.

However, the opening in the capillary wall now also allows entry of the infective agent into the bloodstream for travel into other areas of the body. Cancer cells can also enter the same portals for travel to new destinations through the bloodstream, or exit the bloodstream using the welcoming signals from the inflamed location.

Thus, inflammation, regardless of its cause, can result in not only the production but also the spread of cancer beyond the immediate environment. In fact, just as law enforcement officers and trained emergency medical technicians come to the aid of accident victims, immune cells, not knowing the true identity of cancer cells, may produce similar signaling molecules to promote the formation of new blood vessels and recruit cells, including those from the immune system, to facilitate their movement and settlement in the vicinity of a site of inflammation.

## CURIOUS TIDBITS

The process of a specific immune response of sufficient strength can take up to two weeks or more to mount. This is why you are commonly advised to take preventive immunizations at least two weeks before the expected exposure to an infective agent such as a virus.

# How chronic accelerated cell regeneration is a cause of mutations

A critical factor that explains why cancer increases with age could be the need for frequent cell replacement. I consider this mechanism an important element in my recommendations for how to survive after you have been diagnosed or treated for cancer.

For example, 77 percent of cancers are diagnosed in people age 55 and older. This suggests clearly that long-term cell life plays a role in the development of cancer. As we age, we experience more cell multiplications and increasing exposure to environmental agents, raising the risk of gene mutations that can lead to cancer. This explains why 90 percent of human cancers arise in cells that line the organs and cavities of the body and in cells covering the body, because they experience substantial wear and tear as we age. (The rest of cancers occur in the organs and tissues in between the linings or in cells in the blood and lymph.)

For instance, cells lining the intestine are exposed to digestive enzymes and also experience shearing by food debris during the act of contraction and expansion to move food. These cells are replaced almost daily compared to skin cells that last weeks before being replaced due to stress, strain, and scratches. Similarly, in addition to experiencing shearing with each contraction of muscles to expel urine, cells lining the urinary tract are also susceptible to injury from chemicals filtered out of the blood or infectious agents.

The importance of cell regeneration in cancer formation is made even clearer given the fact that heart muscle cells seldom divide after we are born and rarely develop tumors. Nerve cells almost never divide and do not develop cancer. (Brain cancers arise from cells supporting nerve cells, not the nerve cells themselves.)

## CURIOUS TIDBITS

If the probability of cancer cell formation is identical at each cell division across different species, then, all else being equal, an individual with a large body size should be more prone to cancers than one with smaller body size, simply because the larger size individual would have a larger number of cells and therefore more cells multiplying that could experience damage to genes. However, cancer incidence does not follow this theoretical possibility. For example, the incidence of cancer in elephants, which can weigh up to 4800 kg (10,582 lbs), is almost half the incidence of cancer in humans, despite the fact that elephants have many more fast-growing cells than humans. Young elephants gain more than 1 kg (2.2 lbs) of weight per day until their first birthday. And female elephants reproduce offspring throughout their lifespan of 50 to 80 years and therefore continually have growth-promoting hormones available to enhance cancer cell growth. Yet the incidence of cancer in elephants is not correspondingly high. The elephant cells appear to be twice as sensitive to DNA damage-induced apoptosis as human cells, and that apoptosis prevents mutations from spreading to future cell generations.[19]

# Chronic cell regeneration: Ideal for the initiation and survival of cancer

Here's how a normal cell can become cancerous. Imagine cells lining your intestine getting damaged due to an infection. Some existing stem cells multiply to replace cells that are lost.

Then during the formation of new cells, the non-availability of key nutrients, incorporation of defective nutrients, or the presence of bacterial products can lead to the production of altered genes in some of the newly created cells. More mutations happen as the process continues.

Then let's say a few of these cells are destroyed due to chemicals you inadvertently consumed. These may have entered the food chain from the soil, or were sprayed on crops during cultivation. Or they may have been introduced during processing, or intentionally added during packaging to increase shelf life, enhance flavor or improve appearance. The chemicals could also be due to degradation during storage, from contamination with mold, introduced during processing, preserving, or generated during cooking.

In other cases, chemicals may have been released into the food you are eating from their container, which was made of chemicals—plastic, for example—and subjected to heat as in microwaving to cook or warm them. The presence of oil or fat in the food can facilitate retention of many chemicals released by the container and their entry into the body when you eat. In some instances, chemicals circulating in the bloodstream may have entered the body through the air we breathe, absorbed through the skin from what we came in contact with, or as part of a medical treatment. No matter how the chemicals got there, let's say that while the new cells were generating to replace dead ones, a few chemical-induced mutations occurred.

Then sometime later, you had a viral infection that caused intestinal upset. Again, new cells were produced, and these had additional mutations. Another time, you experienced diarrhea and even some bleeding from the gut due to intolerance to some food you ate or a poison present in it. More new cells are created and some of those acquire additional mutations.

During all this time, let's say your intestine has also been exposed to radiation, either as part of a medical procedure or through environmental exposure, adding even more mutations. Eventually, as the intestinal cells go through these cycles of death and regeneration, they are also exposed to damage caused by free radicals released during normal metabolic activities. And as you age, one or more of these scenarios could have been repeated at random.

In addition, any chronic bacterial infection such as *helicobacter pylori* (H. pylori), can lead to chronic accelerated cell regeneration and eventually cancer. Chronic infection with parasites such as *Schistosoma* is associated with bladder cancer, and that from liver flukes with cancer of the bile duct.

These mutations, in either one particular gene or many genes, can mount up and have a lasting influence on cell activity, and ultimately lead to cancerous cells.

# The link between elevated blood glucose level and cancer

There is no doubt that our increased exposure to cancer-causing agents in the environment causes mutations. Air pollution, for example, may result in increased cases of not only lung cancer but also increased gastrointestinal cancers as we eat pollutants in and on our food.

Some might believe the increase in cancers simply reflects more efficient detection methods and/or the increased ability to diagnose tumors that were too small to be detected earlier. That may account for some of the increases, but there is also an increase in cancers detected in India and in Latin American countries, where advanced technologies to detect cancer have not been readily available to the population at large. This suggests that better detection does not completely explain the rise in cancer cases, although aging and obesity could explain some.

Let me suggest another possibility. Currently there are 20 million people diagnosed with Type 2 diabetes and over 85 million diagnosed with prediabetes in the United States. In China, there are 100 million diagnosed with Type 2 diabetes. That number in India is over 60 million. Studies show that people with Type 2 diabetes are twice as likely to develop certain types of cancer as those without diabetes. This means that the next epidemic to afflict the above-mentioned countries would be that of cancer, unless the incidence of diabetes can be reduced.

Type 2 diabetes is considered a problem caused by insulin resistance. I do not believe, as stated in my book *Eat, Chew, Live*, that humans are evolving to become insulin resistant, just as it is unlikely that humans are evolving to have more gene mutations. Rather I suggest that Type 2 diabetes is a condition related to the consumption of grains and grain-flour products, which produce the greatest amount of glucose that cancer cells depend on to survive and multiply. In nearly all countries where Type 2 diabetes is spreading, grains are currently or are becoming a major portion of the national diet. In the USA, it is wheat and in China and India, it is rice.

This fact is especially critical for people with Type 2 diabetes. Studies show a very strong association between Type 2 diabetes and the incidence of cancer, especially liver and pancreatic cancers, often diagnosed in the same individual.[20] This is not a coincidence; both these organs play a role in metabolizing carbohydrates and have extensive exposure to elevated glucose and insulin levels. The liver is the organ through which all glucose from the intestine after meals must pass. The pancreas is responsible for releasing insulin in response to elevated blood glucose levels. Therefore, any cancer cell appearing in these two organs will be the beneficiary of easily available glucose. In addition, the risk for colorectal, breast, urinary tract, and endometrial cancers is also increased in patients with high blood sugar levels.

In short, the rising incidence of cancer is linked to the rising incidence of obesity and Type 2 diabetes—and all are linked to the consumption of grains in excess of what our forefathers consumed, in terms of percentage of energy consumed during a meal. Aging and coming into contact with environmental pollutants may be increasingly relevant contributory factors for cancer that you cannot avoid, but avoiding the consumption of grains and grain-flour products is clearly one choice you *can* make.

# Insulin as a cancer stimulant

Many studies show that people with Type 2 diabetes have a greater chance of developing many types of cancers compared to those without the disease. A study over seven years involving over 70,000 women aged 40-70 showed a high carbohydrate diet to be positively associated with breast cancer risk in premenopausal women.[21] Diabetes appears to be associated with substantial premature mortality from several cancers.[22]

While glucose feeds cancer cells, insulin released from the pancreas in response to blood sugar elevation helps cancer cell multiplication. Thus, diabetics who stimulate the pancreas with a medication, or who inject insulin into the body, could actually be stimulating the growth of any cancer cell in the body. By binding to a receptor on the cell surface, insulin initiates a signal that travels to the cell nucleus, resulting in the stimulation of genes that produce proteins essential for cell division. This encourages cell multiplication.

In today's typical heavy carbohydrate western diet—three meals per day plus occasional snacks and/or drinks also containing carbohydrates—most people have elevated insulin levels nearly all day long.

In addition to being a signal for growth, insulin can induce the formation of enzymes needed for glycolysis, to extract energy from glucose. Insulin also appears to inhibit cellular "stickiness," so cancer cells get more freedom to move out of their tumor mass. For example, in one study, cultured cancer cells exhibited the following behavior. When blood glucose concentration is at the level often found in Type 2 diabetes, cancer cells from breast, colon, prostate, and bladder not only multiplied faster but also showed more rapid movement indicating the potential for cancer spread.[23] Even more ominous was the finding that the addition of insulin to a high-glucose environment enhanced cancer cell multiplication by 20-40%. And finally, when elevated blood sugar levels persist for a long time, cancer cells are found to increase their multiplication rate.[24]

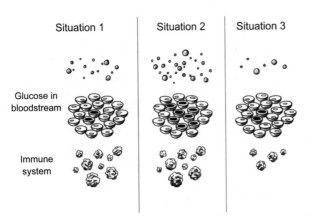

Situation 1    Situation 2    Situation 3

Glucose in bloodstream

Immune system

By and large, the amount of glucose absorbed, largely from grain products you eat, will influence the progression of cancer. In Situation 1, if you have very little glucose in your bloodstream and a normal immune system, cancer cells will find it difficult to grow. In Situation 2, if you have a high level of glucose in your bloodstream, cancer cell growth may occur even if you have a normal immune system. Situation 3 shows that if you have a weakened immune system, you can control cancer growth by maintaining low normal glucose in your bloodstream.

# Detecting cancer and the most common treatments

IT IS IMPORTANT TO RECOGNIZE THAT WHILE MUTATIONS ARE INherited by successive generations of cancer cells, the order of those gene mutations is less important than their total accumulation. As the cancer progresses, subpopulations of cancer cells can differ in the type of mutations, physical appearance, rate of growth, invasiveness, responsiveness to growth promoters, and the susceptibility to antineoplastic drugs. Therefore, it is important to understand as much as we can about each type of cancer to decide potentially the most effective treatment strategy.

In general, a treatment strategy is first tested in a laboratory setting. This often involves growing cancer cells in cultures and exposing some of them to an agent or condition and looking for the effect, such as inhibiting the rate of growth relative to similar cancer cells not exposed to the same agent or condition.

The next step is to test the method in an animal study. Here the animal is first rendered incapable of fighting cancer by incapacitating its own immune system. Then known cancer cells are injected or implanted into the test animals, making sure of their growth. Some are then exposed to the agent or condition to be tested, just as in the cell culture, keeping some similar animals with cancer as controls.

There are limitations to such tests, though. It could arise that the positive results in a culture of cancer cells may not be duplicated in the animal study. Or the results of the cell culture or the animal study may not be duplicated in a human being.

# A growing array of early testing methods for cancer susceptibility

Detection of cancer susceptibility before cancer is established, or detection of cancer in its early stages, is clearly helpful to prevent it or eradicate it from the body. This is a growing focus of scientific research. Such greater understanding can help target for treatment any molecules inside cancer cells that are responsible for abnormal multiplication.

Many tests are currently on the market to determine your susceptibility to different types of cancer. Here are some of the tests:

- Some cancers, even in the early stages, leave markers, such as proteins or bits of genes containing telltale signs of cancer that have been released into body fluids and found their way into the bloodstream (e.g., Alpha-fetoprotein in liver cancer). Periodic search for such markers could lead to early detection of cancer already present in people over 55 and those who have identifiable cancer risk.

- Screening blood samples for the presence of cancer cells or cancer DNA can identify patients having a specific cancer (e.g., abnormal lymphocytes in leukemia). Similar tests may also identify those who have a higher than normal susceptibility to specific cancers.

- Some tumors can be detected by looking for signs of their high production of energy. Using special molecules similar to glucose that have been "tagged," doctors can detect their absorption by cancer cells using radiological testing (such as a PET scan in tumor imaging).

- Another testing methodology examines genes to reveal not only the presence of cancer, but also how aggressive it is (e.g., single-nucleotide polymorphism). This can help guide the decision to wait watchfully or begin immediate treatment. However, in order to analyze and test actual genes, one has to have access to a cell that can be examined in the laboratory. Some locations, such as the ovary, are difficult to get samples from. By the time a cancer is detected, it may already be too late to destroy all the cancer cells using currently available means. Efforts are underway to find better detection procedures for cancers in bodily areas that are hard to sample.

The best examples of successful early screening tests are the Pap smear that can detect malignant changes in the outer layer of the cervix, and mammography, which can detect cancer before it starts the invasion process in the breast.

Note that you have to make sure of the validity of these tests to determine your susceptibility to cancer and your options as to what to do. For example, results of similar tests using tissue samples from the same patient done in two different laboratories may disagree.

# Problems in cancer screening

As stated earlier, solid cancers require between 20 and 30 generational doublings before they attain a clinically detectable size over durations of many years.[25] By the time the number of doublings reaches 40, extensive disease is present. After another few doublings, death usually ensues.

In the future, as individuals undergo more screening, such as looking for proteins involved with the formation of new blood vessels (vascular endothelial growth factor VEGF), ingesting fluorescent molecules that attach to cancer cells to make them more visible, or identifying specific proteins released by cancer cells, cancers that might be too small to cause problems may be detected and treatments offered.

Meanwhile, the current downside of cancer knowledge is that many tests are expensive. In addition, the results can be confusing. This can often put individuals under strain to decide which is the most appropriate course of action when 100 percent certainty is still lacking.

Some testing is also "irrelevant" compared to a person's lifetime. For example, prostate cancer screening based on prostate-specific antigen (PSA) testing increases cancer detection but it may not impact mortality. PSA is an enzyme present in small quantities in the serum of men with healthy prostates, but is often elevated in the presence of prostate cancer or other prostate disorders. But there is an important controversy with PSA screening for prostate cancer—sometimes a person's life expectancy is actually lower than the time frame in which cancer would become clinically meaningful, raising the question: is it appropriate to treat or even screen that person?

Testing for cancer is also complicated by the fact that not all gene mutations result in cancer. One way to get around this dilemma is to identify the protein signal that is ultimately responsible for cell division and trace it back to the gene producing the first signaling molecule. Researchers are therefore developing lines of cells with genes from only one parent to study the role of specific mutation in cancer initiation and progression, because removal of the normal working copy of the same gene could force the mutant gene to express.

In addition, the use of a PET scan to detect the presence of cancer could be complicated by excessive metabolic activity at a site of inflammation. Because of this, not all positive PET scans imply cancer, and not all negative tests suggest absence of cancer.

# The current capabilities in testing for genetic mutations

There are many known cancer predisposition genes. Inheritance of these increases the risk that a person may develop cancer. Clearly, identifying these gene mutations will allow early detection of the potential for cancer.

The most well-known of these is the mutated gene(s) that is overexpressed in breast, ovarian, stomach, uterine, and some lung cancers. For example, breast cancer can be divided into subtypes based on gene expression. Most human breast cancer occurs in women with no known predisposition, but about 10 percent of breast cancers are associated with inherited defects in two genes, BRCA1 and BRCA2. Women with these damaged genes have a greater than 80% chance of developing breast cancer. In certain populations, such as Ashkenazi Jews, up to 1% of the women may have mutations in these genes, though the reason is unknown.

It is becoming increasingly possible to visualize the genes and molecular structures within cancer cells. For example, with the use of a process called the *polymerase chain reaction* (PCR), a single piece of genetic material can be used to create millions of copies. This test is currently employed to do leukemia and lymphoma classification.

However, screening for gene mutations to target a specific cancer for identification and treatment may prove problematic because fast-growing cancer cells can exhibit other mutations than the parent cell of the cancer. For example, it is not uncommon to have 50 mutations in breast, pancreas, and brain cancers. Thus, treatment that eliminates cells with one type of gene mutation may not remove cancer cells that have another type of mutation.

Furthermore, identifying the type of gene mutation during a first episode of cancer does not mean that the same will apply to a recurrence years later, because the second cancer could be due to subsequent mutations that are different from the first.

## CURIOUS TIDBITS

When completed, the Cancer Genome Atlas will show how many mutated genes exist in each cancer. This may make it possible to detect gene mutations that can be compared with those who had cancer to calculate one's cancer susceptibility of, say, lung cancer.

However, variations in genetics that occur due to the appearance of new genes in a population as a result of interbreeding or population change after any genetic data has been collected may skew future conclusions. The Atlas also does not guarantee that an individual will have only those mutations throughout the life of that cancer or that the mutations will be identical in two people diagnosed with the same cancer.

# More on detecting genetic mutations

Although specific gene alterations vary between different cancer types, defects in genome maintenance and repair have been detected in the great majority of human cancers. Increased exposure or sensitivity to mutagenic agents, breakdown of one or several components of a gene maintenance system, a compromised surveillance mechanism—all these can result in genetic mutations.

Altered genes signal they have cancer potential by producing proteins that physically resemble normal proteins made by the same cells, but without the same functionality. It may seem smart to attempt to detect gene mutations before they reach that cancer threshold, especially in people who may have an inherited genetic susceptibility. At present, there is a method to do that using ultrasensitive digitalized protein detection that uncovers subtle but important differences in signaling by cancer cells.[26] But not all cancers produce these telltale proteins, thyroid cancer being an example.

In addition, although this test has proven to be helpful to detect proteins in a known cancer cell, its usefulness to identify cancer lacks certainty for many reasons. First, which cell in the target organ or tissue should one look at? How often should the test be conducted? Is it possible to detect an accelerated rate of multiplication of a particular cell line? Only future research will tell.

In short, it can be difficult to detect cancer. Keep in mind that cell multiplication can become exaggerated due to enhanced signaling at different points in the signaling cascade. Early detection of mutations in each and every one of these points in the human body through laboratory testing is not dependable at this time.

Enhanced gene mutations, especially in the later stages of cancer progression, can also result in the creation of subpopulations of cancer cells that may become more resistant to chemotherapy, remain dormant for years or even decades, or create subpopulations that multiply more rapidly than they can be eliminated. Even more baffling is the possibility of cancer cells acquiring gene mutations that enable them to metamorphose into supporting cells or cells that can form new blood vessels or lymphatic channels that serve as migration conduits.

# The three primary cancer treatments: surgery, radiation, and chemotherapy

## Surgery

Removing cancer cells by surgery has been practiced for a long time. Surgery works best if the cancer growth is localized and accessible, such as in the testicles where it's possible to surgically remove the entire testicle. Surgery can also work indirectly to remove something that bolsters the cancer cells, such as removing the ovaries to starve breast cancer cells that are hormone sensitive. When considering surgery, ask these questions:

- How will surgery impact survival and quality of life?
- Do you need chemotherapy and/or radiation in addition to surgery? If so, will that make a difference in survival and quality of life?
- Are there specific steps to prevent recurrence of the cancer?

## Radiation

Soon after x-rays were first invented in the laboratory, it was discovered that the energy from a penetrating x-ray could cause significant damage to the inner structure of cancer cells, resulting in their death. However, some cancer cells can develop robust self-repair mechanisms that quickly repair their own gene mutations and tolerate radiation. In addition, caution has to be exercised because radiation of sufficient magnitude can result in causing gene mutations in the surrounding tissue, which might trigger a different type of cancer in the formerly non-cancerous cells.

## Chemotherapy

Although in some cases chemical agents can be administered directly into a tumor, chemotherapy is often administered when the cancer is not localized and cannot be destroyed by targeted treatment using radiation or surgery. In such cases, using drugs to kill the cancer cells is one of the most common methods of treating cancer, either alone or sometimes in conjunction with surgery, radiation, hormones, or immunological therapy.

Note, however, chemotherapy has some drawbacks. It can affect other rapidly dividing cells such as red blood cells, resulting in anemia. If the chemical impacts white blood cells, it can result in a reduced ability to fight infection. If the chemical causes reduced platelets, it can result in decreased ability to form a clot.

In addition, some chemotherapy medications may inhibit the growth of rapidly dividing cells in the hair follicles, mouth, skin, and the intestine. This can cause discomfort or more serious health problems.

# How does chemotherapy work?

Certain chemicals are capable of causing a gene mutation. When repeated exposures to such chemicals result in uncontrolled multiplication of a cell, the chemical is called a carcinogen. But when exposure to chemicals can damage cell structures to the point of being unable to carry on cellular function, the cell dies. This is called chemotherapy.

A targeted chemotherapy treatment starts with identifying a vulnerable target in the specific area of the cancer. Any chemical that can interfere with the maturation, multiplication, or migration of cancer cells can be used as the therapeutic agent. Some drugs can be given into the vein, others are swallowed, and still others are injected into the body. These can reach all parts of the body through the bloodstream.

However, there is a potential for resistance to develop with chemotherapy. Cancer cells can develop internal mechanisms to resist or bypass the effect of chemical agents. Or chemotherapy can affect cells in and around the cancer, prompting them to produce protein molecules that resist the chemotherapy. The rapid identification of the mechanism(s) of resistance, if available, can potentially overcome such resistance.

In addition, chemotherapy can inhibit surveillance by immune cells on common viruses and bacteria. For example, viruses such as hepatitis B and chicken pox, and tuberculosis bacteria that have been kept under control may be reactivated when the immune system is impacted. This can cause reactivation and infection in the host. In rare cases, chemotherapy intended to kill cancer cells of one variety may result in the formation of a different type of cancer. For example, while reducing the risk of breast cancer in women, the drug tamoxifen may increase the risk of endometrial cancer.

Finally, chemotherapy may not completely eradicate cancer because of mutated stem cells that are yet to function fully. Every healthy tissue has Phase 2 stem cells that can produce the specific tissue cells. If your cancer has Phase 2 stem cells that were not eradicated by the chemotherapy treatment, they could be reactivated under appropriate stimulus to produce cancer cells.

# Other common cancer treatments

## Cryosurgery

Use of extreme cold, as in cryosurgery, has been commonly used to treat some types of cancer, especially that of the skin. The cold is applied to skin areas using frozen nitrogen gas.

## Laser

Laser beams can be used to cut tissue. For example, very small cancers of the stomach without lymph node involvement can be effectively treated with lasers. Esophageal cancers that obstruct the passage of food into the stomach can be trimmed with laser surgery. The same procedure can be used to relieve bowel obstructions in colorectal cancer.

## Biosurgery

One of the newest treatments is biosurgery, in which specially modified bacteria that survive in an oxygen-free environment and release cancer-killing enzymes are injected into a solid tumor to destroy it. The bacteria work against cancer because cancer cells often contain reduced oxygen levels, called hypoxia. Reduced oxygen actually helps tumor cells resist cancer treatment by radiation because radiation treatment uses free radicals from oxygen to destroy its target cells. Reduced oxygen inside solid tumors also facilitates the production of a variety of agents that help form new blood vessels.

Fortunately, after poisoning and killing cancer cells, when the bacteria encounter oxygen molecules in the normal tissue, they themselves are destroyed, eliminating the prospect of an infection in the patient.

In addition, products of the bacteria may enhance the person's normal immune response with not only destruction of the cancer cells but also in building immunity to other diseases. It now seems that combining this type of biosurgery with other cancer therapies can result in better outcomes.

## Proton beam therapy

One way to disable mutated genes from functioning is to damage their molecular structure at the atomic level. This is what happens during proton beam therapy that removes electrons from DNA molecules, making them unable to issue instructions for cell multiplication. Proton beams can be more focused, not much larger in size than the eraser on a pencil, resulting in less collateral damage compared to some other forms of radiation therapy.

# Additional cancer treatments in early trials

## Photodynamic therapy

Some tumor tissue takes up the photosensitizer *Photophrin II* when it is administered into the body. Subsequent exposure to laser causes the production of highly toxic substances with resultant death of cancer cells. This is currently used in gastrointestinal tract and bronchial cancers.

## Oncolytic virotherapy

Researchers are devising ways to genetically alter viruses to kill cancer cells with minimum unwanted side effects. Viruses can be trained to selectively enter cancer cells, hijack those cells' gene-copying faculties and direct production of new copies of themselves. They can burst out of the cancer cell looking for similar cells hiding anywhere in the body and repeat the action until no more cancer cells remain. When no more cancer cells are available these viruses die for lack of a suitable host cell.

This has many advantages. While many cancer drugs interfere with only one aspect of cell functioning, viruses disrupt many processes in the cell all at once. Even when all cancer cells descend from a common ancestor, mutations during subsequent multiplication can lead to many different types of cancer cells. However, viruses have the ability to enter cancer cells with an identifiable outside marker they are trained to look for.

However, one limiting factor of virotherapy is that it might cause an immune response directed against the virus. On the other hand, the immune cells may also attack cancer cells harboring viruses just as they do during any viral infection.

## Other therapies

Another tactic is to counter the driving force of the cancer. For example, if the cancer depends on a normal biological agent such as testosterone, opposing the action of the hormone using estrogen can execute a sort of "chemical castration" and arrest its progress, at least until the cancer develops resistance. Another example is using a synthetic female hormone with the structural similarities to, but not the functional capabilities of, estrogen that enable it to be accepted by cancer cells, which then are unable to turn on their multiplication process. The medication tamoxifen works in this fashion. Using inhibitors of growth-promoting molecular agents released during inflammation is another method in the prevention and treatment of cancer.

In general, clinical trials are the gold standard for testing the efficacy of new therapies. However, many of these exclude elderly, frail, or socially disadvantaged people. So, the results may not be applicable on a global basis. Population-based survival studies are needed that include all patients—young and old, rich and poor, with early or late disease, and with or without comorbidity, not just the small percentage of younger, fitter patients typically recruited for clinical trials.

# Using gene manipulation to stop cancer

There are several methods of manipulating genes to stop cancer. In one, the gene is intentionally mutated to prevent cell multiplication. The chemical *cisplantin* ties up the two strands of a gene, making it impossible for them to separate to create proteins needed for multiplication. Although every cell can be potentially impacted, those cells that are actively dividing, such as cancer cells are affected the most.

Unfortunately, as the use of cisplantin to treat many cancers became more common, so did the emergence of resistance to its action. Cancer cells are able to do this in many ways, including: decreased attachment of the drug to receptors on the cancer cell wall, increased detoxification of the drug, not listening to the signal that is supposed to initiate the self-death program, and making rapid repairs to the gene damage.

Some other drugs can shut down how cancer cells function. For example, people with HER2 mutations can have many more receptors on their cancer cells that respond to growth-stimulating signals. The drug *trastuzumab* neutralizes that type of breast cancer by shutting down those receptors. Combining a trastuzumab molecule with a chemotherapeutic agent makes the drug even more effective. Similarly, the drug *sunitinib* can halt a specific type of leukemia. Also in use now are inhibitors of specific enzymes that fuel cell growth, such as in lung cancer associated with people who have never smoked.

Introducing agents that can enter a targeted cancer cell and change mutated genes is another method. In the same way that the hepatitis virus enters a liver cell, researchers may be able to insert agents that change mutated genes that have the propensity to multiply uncontrollably. This will slow the growth of cancer cells.

Inhibiting any one of the critical signaling pathways from the gene, such as interfering with the function of the specific kinase, is also another method. This could stop the signaling process to multiply, at least until or unless the cancer cell develops another mutation to overcome that interference.

Glucose inhibitors may be used to block the functional capability of hyperactive genes. Glucose molecules tagged with anticancer agents could be viable against very rapidly multiplying cells.

However, the challenge in gene manipulation is when there are multiple mutations in a gene. Since multiple mutations may be present in a single type of cancer, it means that we need more targeted therapy to ensure that each mutation is being counteracted in the right way.

# The future of gene manipulation

Many new methods are being investigated that relate to gene manipulation. Here is an overview of some of them:

### Cutting off the mutated part of a gene

Researchers have learned to tame a natural process used by bacteria to cut the genetic materials of viruses that invade cells. One day this technique could become available to cut off the mutated or malfunctioning part of a gene. The cell's normal repair program can then replace the mutated part as it is trained to do. However, unlike a surgeon who can cut the immediate normal cells surrounding the mass and remove it totally while not touching a similar site in a duplicate organ in the body, kidney or breast for example, the biological scissor may not allow for such discrimination.

There are significant differences in DNA mutations between the original tumor and metastasis. However, if the signaling coming from the original cancer is needed for the survival of new cancer cells, then removal of that may terminate not only the original cancer but also the satellites.

### Using microRNA

As explained in the section "How genes control the function of cells," micro RNAs aid in the transcription of information contained in genes. So it is not surprising to find them helping the activity of cancer genes. However, in a normal cell, another micro RNA shuts down the transcription. Identification of the specific micro RNA that shuts down the transcription in a cancer cell could open up new immunological treatments. Similarly, drugs could target the specific messenger proteins to slow the progression of cancer.

### Engineering stem cells to destroy cancer

A stem cell can be equipped like a heat-seeking missile with specific sensors to reach protein markers on a particular cancer cell. The warhead carried by the stem cell will be an enzyme that can convert a nontoxic medication, called a prodrug, that is taken separately, into an active cell-killing agent. This means that only cells having the tumor-specific protein on the surface will be killed, sparing normal cells because normal cells lack the enzyme needed to activate the prodrug. Stem cells can also be loaded with specific cancer-killing viruses engineered to produce proteins that inhibit tumor growth and injected into the body to destroy almost any kind of cancer.

Ordinarily, everyone has sentinel lymphocytes that can recognize cancer cells by the presence of identification proteins on the wall and launch an attack to kill them. However, certain cancers can use the attachment of killer cells on their proteins to keep them in place so that these cells act as a shield to block attacks from other agents or killer cells. Blocking this type of attachment is an area of interest as a potential cancer therapy.

# Immunotherapy to combat cancer

The primary objective of immunotherapy is to shore up your body's natural defenses against cancer, similar to what happens when your body has been invaded by a bacteria or virus. Agents of the immune system are released in large numbers and begin scouting the body to detect invaders and inform the regional lymph node to mount an attack to eliminate them. Some of the unexplained cures of cancer experienced by patients could be of this nature, though credited to miraculous healing or some other non-scientific explanation.

Immune manipulation for cancer can take many different forms, from attacking the mutated gene(s), to blocking the signal transmission that supports cancer cell resistance to chemotherapeutic agents, to disarming or killing cancer cells. Formulating a therapy based on a specific cancer type could help develop opportunities for more targeted and effective treatments. It could also help reduce the strength of the chemotherapy, which could lessen its numerous uncomfortable side effects.

Some of the methods of immunotherapy, both in research and practice, are:

1.  Scientists can harvest a patient's immune cells, select those with the best tumor fighting capabilities and grow them in the laboratory to increase their density. They are then injected back into the patient in an attempt to kill cancer cells. This can be very useful if a sufficient number of these cells can be grown safely and economically. They can roam the body looking for and killing cancer cells without destroying normal ones and without provoking an immune response against them by the body.

2.  *Sipulencel-T* in conjunction with a helper molecule exposes a patient's own white blood cells to proteins extracted from the cancer cells of the patient. After training, these white cells are infused back into the patient to fight cancer.[27] In some cases, new genes can be inserted into the lymphocytes before infusing them back into the body. The modified lymphocytes would then multiply inside the body to produce an army of killer cells that are trained to destroy cancer cells. Additionally, these reengineered killer cells may live for many years in the body policing the formation of new cancer cells.

## More on immunotherapy

Since cancer means abnormal growth driven by a normal gene gone haywire or on overdrive, identifying such genes and blocking the production of proteins they command can be an effective way to stop cancer in its tracks.

However, unlike humans, many single cell organisms have redundant pathways to repair gene damages. If cancer cells acquire this capability, they could develop resistance to therapeutic agents that work that way.

On the other hand, inhibiting gene signaling can be effective in cancers having the same gene mutation regardless of the types of cells in the body, and thus they can be treated with a similar drug. In this way, getting a better understanding of the common molecular pattern of genetic changes can help in treating cancers using the same chemotherapeutic agents or other specific measures to disable the responsible gene regardless of the organ, such as breast and ovary, in which cancer is located.

In order to become a part of an organ or tissue, a stem cell has to keep active genes necessary to perform its designated function, while switching off genes that make it a stem cell. However, some cancer cells mutate back to activate genes needed to function as a stem cell so that they can restart multiplication and become cancerous. Identifying and blocking this functionality is another form of immune therapy.

# Stimulating the body's immune system

The body may activate defense mechanisms consisting of antibodies, killer cells, and even increased local temperature to slow down unwanted cell multiplication. There are also ways to trigger the body's own immune system to function more aggressively. These include:

- infusing the body with agents to elicit an inflammatory response that can mobilize killer cells
- infusing the body with antibodies against cancer cells, by themselves or coupled with a toxin capable of killing the cancer cells

Studies are also underway on ways to prevent cancer from coming back by administering a vaccine made from a patient's own cancer cells to provoke an immune response.[28]

## Other trials

For many infections, it is a common procedure to grow bacteria from the patient in a laboratory and test antibiotics to find the one that works best to kill them. In the same way, it is possible to grow cancer cells in the lab and test them against various chemotherapy agents to detect the best one for that type of cancer. In fact, almost all cancer drugs in current use were first tested against cultured cells in a laboratory.

In addition to manipulation of the immune system for a specific cancer, researchers are also exploring non-specific avenues. An example is experiments using bacterial agents injected into the body that activate the immune system and result in controlling or even eliminating cancer cells from the body, at least for a while. However, it has not yet been shown that this approach can eliminate cancer on a long-term basis.

Another promising avenue of therapy is identifying the mechanism by which cancer cells avoid activation of the self-destruct sequence leading to their own death. Interfering with how cancer cells achieve this mode of survival is a possible treatment.

## Risks

Manipulating the immune system to suppress cancer carries the danger of making it hyper-vigilant to the point of launching an autoimmune response and its consequences. In addition, one has to be aware of collateral damages. For example, attacking cancer cells in bone marrow can harm normal cells, leading to interference with critical functions in the body. Since cancer cells use the same methodology as normal cells to multiply, whatever action we take to prevent or slow down cancer formation may impact the function of normal cells too.

# More methods of stimulating the body's immune system

1.  Blood supply is the most important factor in the rate of cancer growth because oxygen and nutrients needed by a cell cannot reach over a distance of 1 to 2 mm. As explained earlier, cancer cells may release vascular endothelial growth factor (VEGF), which stimulates the growth of blood vessels to facilitate grabbing a bigger share of nutrients. A receptor called vascular endothelial growth factor receptor (VEGFR) must be activated for the formation of new blood vessels to provide a solid cancer with its own blood supply. Inhibitors of VEGFR could prove valuable in the treatment of cancer. However, these agents should not inhibit the formation of beneficial blood vessels.

2.  Some cancers may have proteins on the surface of their cells capable of responding to growth promoters to fuel their growth. In such cases, blocking the promoter from attaching to the proteins may slow the cancer cells from multiplying. For instance, the female hormone estrogen fuels the growth and spread of breast cancer. Medications that block the synthesis of estrogen could prevent the recurrence of breast cancer. However, estrogen also inhibits cells that cause osteoporosis. Thus, blockage of estrogen could lead to the formation of brittle bones and bone fractures.

3.  Killer cells activated by proteins from a cancer cell may continue to attack any cell having similar identification badges, similar to an autoimmune response. To prevent this, nature has an inhibitor built into newly formed killer cells. However, if the inhibitor is activated too early, it might prevent complete elimination of cancer cells. Therefore, blocking the inhibitor of killer cells, until their job is completed, is another form of immune therapy.

Note: Since most laboratories are used by multiple researchers and employ many technicians, procedures should be in place so that lines of cancer cells do not become contaminated by one another. It is especially disruptive to research if there are cancer cells that can grow at different rates in the same culture medium. This can cause problems that may not be detected unless cancer researchers periodically test to verify the purity of their cancer cell lines. Without such safeguards, drugs may be tested against the wrong cancer cells and found not useful, or the researcher may get false positive results, or cell cultures may lead to erroneous conclusions about the very nature of the development of cancer.

Compounding this is the potential for cancer cells to mutate in the laboratory environment. With proper safeguards in place, growing cancer cells from each patient in a laboratory, identifying the specific genetic mutations, and rating the aggressiveness of growth can help narrow the selection of drug(s) for treating each cancer.

# Using high temperature to kill cancer

Human cancer cells are more readily destroyed by hyperthermia (higher than normal body temperature) than regular human cells. But this does not mean that you should crank up the heat. Although humans can stand prolonged exposure to temperatures up to 43 degrees C (109 F), this is not a practical way to restrict the growth of cancer cells.

However, hyperthermia, while yet to be clinically proven, may be useful as an adjunct to chemotherapy or radiotherapy with improved results. Cancer cells that thrive in an environment of low oxygen are normally resistant to radiation, but they appear to lose some resistance when experiencing hyperthermia. The same is true for chemotherapy.

Another instance where hyperthermia can be immediately useful in cancer treatment is when a patient's bone marrow has been harvested prior to radiation, to be infused back into the patient after the treatment. Hyperthermia treatment of the harvested bone marrow may kill any residual cancer cells in the harvest.

However, even a sustained, significant elevation of the body temperature may not be beneficial with a solid tumor that has built a capsule around it.

# The role of body temperature in cancer formation

A proper physical environment is essential for all cells to grow, especially newly formed ones, whether they are normal or cancerous. This is why the body has a highly responsive temperature regulatory system. When exercising generates a large heat load as a result of muscular work, the regulatory mechanisms kick in to prevent an excessive and potentially dangerous rise in body temperature. This is particularly true in hot, humid conditions, where sweat that may not evaporate quickly enough can result in developing severe hyperthermia.

It is a well-known fact that elevation of the body temperature during an infection by an agent such as a virus is an attempt by the body to slow viral multiplication. In this regard, cancer cells grown in a laboratory are also less tolerant of high temperature, such that hyperthermia may induce the killing of cancer cells.

### CURIOUS TIDBITS

The most visible example of the importance of environmental temperature for the maintenance of cell health is the dangling of the scrotum so that the testes can maintain optimum temperature—2°C below the internal temperature—for sperm development. On very cold days, scrotal muscles contract to bring the testes close to the body to maintain the temperature. Failure of temperature maintenance as happens when one testis remains inside the abdomen of the baby, called undescended testis, or cryptorchidism, causes degeneration leading to impaired fertility. There is then a potential for the generation of damaged testicular cells under hormonal stimulus with the risk of cancer formation, compared to a male with normally descended testes. Surgical correction before the age of 13 appears to significantly ameliorate complications, including the incidence of cancer.[29]

# How to Survive Cancer

Cancer survivability is high if it can be prevented from spreading. According to a 2014 report from the American Cancer Society, deaths from all types of cancer for both men and women are estimated to peak between the ages 40 and 65 years. Using current statistics, the chance of succumbing to cancer after being diagnosed is 50%. This percentage is too high, and it is what I seek to change for the better in this book, giving you information you need to put your cancer, your treatment, and your ultimate survivability in perspective.

Cancer, Type 2 diabetes, and obesity are considered lifestyle diseases. However, these conditions are seen with increasing frequency in countries such as the United States, China, and India—countries with obviously different lifestyles. So identifying a common lifestyle factor could be useful to deal with all three conditions, regardless of the country you live in or whether you move to a different place.

What is common in these three conditions? The answer is glucose, as this Part will detail. I provide a wide range of actions you can take to keep your diagnosed cancer at bay and prevent cancer cells from spreading to other parts of your body. It includes advice on:

- Starving cancer cells
- What to eat and enjoy
- Weight control, fat loss, and exercise
- Avoiding environmental toxins and pollutants
- Sleep
- Stress-reduction

The above strategies can also be used to prevent cancer recurrence, if you have already had it.

# Starving cancer cells

THE PRESENCE OF NATURAL KILLER CELLS [NK CELLS] SUGGESTS that formation of cancer cells in the body is an expected event even in an immunologically intact individual, and nature has provided the necessary steps to deal with it. Increased occurrence of cancer as we get older suggests the unavoidable nature of genetic mutations as one continues to be exposed to both internal and external causes of gene damage. The finding of cancer remaining dormant for many years suggests that the human body can continue living while being a host to it. The key appears to be preventing the appearance of cancer cells that can resist the existing capabilities of the immune system. The best way to accomplish this is by limiting multiplication of any cancer cell in the body so that new variants that resist immune attack do not emerge.

Cancer cells are formed in the body at random, but the easy availability of glucose promotes their rapid multiplication, overpowering the capabilities of immune cells to destroy them. Since cancer cells don't use fatty acids to produce energy for multiplication, if they are deprived of their preferred fuel, glucose, they starve. In addition to energy, a cancer cell can obtain from glucose molecules the carbon skeletons needed for the fabrication of every amino acid, genetic material, fatty acid, or other metabolic intermediaries needed for growth.

Starving cancer cells is the best course of action to take to survive.

# The key to starving cancer cells

As you learned earlier in the book, cancer cells are driven by the need to survive. They are reverting back to their default mission, returning to what I have called their Adam Cell programming, in which their goal is simply to divide to survive at all costs. In the same way that rapidly dividing embryonic cells use glucose breakdown outside the mitochondria for their energy production, then use the byproducts to manufacture structures and functional intermediaries, cancer cells do the same.

Given this, the most effective opportunity you have to halt the spread of cancer to more territory in its original site of existence, as well as to combat its spread elsewhere in the body, is to prevent the cancer cells from multiplying.

Based on what we know about cancer cells, I am convinced that the best, natural way to accomplish this—regardless of the type, location, size, or age—is to starve them.

Effectively, I am talking about starving cancer cells of glucose, their main source of energy as well as building material. It has been shown that the rate of growth of human cancer cells in mice was slowed when the availability of glucose was restricted, even in mice with a compromised immune system. In effect, *no glucose, no cancer growth.* [30] (Since the liver can make glucose using many agents, what I am suggesting is the restriction of glucose sources that are in our direct control.) Under these conditions, cancer cells will be similar to a gas-guzzler car operating under gas rationing.

Given that cancer cells compete for nutrients with all other cells in their vicinity, the key to control cancer cells is to prevent them from gaining access to nutrients. Cancer cells are focused mostly on multiplying themselves, rather than performing any other cellular functions. As a result, they can forgo acquiring the many other nutrients that normal cells would ordinarily need to function in the tissue they are part of. Therefore, the only significant nutrient cancer cells need and want is glucose—and they excel at stealing it from other cells.

This means the most promising approach to slow down cell multiplication leading to the metastasis of cancer is to deny its primary fuel source—glucose. This is the strategy I am proposing in this book. I believe it is the Achilles' heel of all cancer cells—the need for glucose to survive.

# Cancer cells excel at obtaining glucose

The presence of glucose molecules outside a cell does not mean automatic entry of glucose inside the cell. This is mostly determined by the type of glucose transporters, which, in turn, are determined by the type of cells in the body. Humans are known to have twelve glucose transporters, each with unique properties based on location and function.

For example, red blood cells relying on the dependable glycolysis method of ATP production need a steady supply of glucose. For this purpose, they manufacture GLUT-1 transporters that can facilitate entry of glucose 50,000 times greater than what could enter the cell without help. Glucose transporters associated with liver cells (GLUT-1 and GLUT-2) and brain neurons (GLUT-3) are always present on the cell membrane to catch any glucose molecules passing by. In contrast, the main glucose transporter in muscle cells and fat cells (GLUT-4) is sequestered inside the cell and moves to the cell membrane only in response to a signal transmitted from insulin outside the cell. [31]

Glucose transporters are like little trucks carrying glucose molecules from the cell membrane into the cell. Cancer cells excel at manufacturing glucose transporters, especially those that do not require insulin for activation.

To satisfy their voracious appetite for glucose, cancer cells produce an abundance of two different glucose transporters; these transporters do not require activation by insulin and are capable of catching glucose molecules even when they are in numbers too low to be picked up by insulin-activated transporters.

**CURIOUS TIDBITS**

The abundance of GLUT-1 glucose transporters in the cell membrane of cancer cells helps identify a diverse group of cancers in a Positron Emission Tomography (PET) scan. Elevated glucose metabolism allows detection of the location of cancer, and helps with cancer staging, therapeutic response, and the differentiation of post-therapy changes from residual tumor.[32]

# Why cancer cells might die without glucose for their fuel

In many types of cancer cells found in humans, malignant melanoma, for example, glucose uptake and the breakdown of glucose into ATP (glycolysis) proceed about 10 times faster than in a normal cell.

Why is this? Since cancer cells do not have functioning mitochondria they are unable to generate ATP using the more efficient oxygen-dependent process that utilizes fatty acids. Instead, cancer cells must rely on glucose to create all their energy *outside* of the mitochondria.

As a result, cancer cells go after glucose voraciously. In fact, cancer cells undergo a real feeding frenzy soon after a meal when glucose is abundant. Ordinarily, the fluid around cells contains 75 – 95 milligrams per deciliter (mg/dl) of glucose on average. However, in the period immediately after a meal, the blood glucose level can go up to 1500 mg/dl without any untoward consequences to the body. This creates an excellent opportunity for cancer cells to load up on glucose.

Indeed, many statistics appear to show a strong correlation between excess glucose in your bloodstream (high blood sugar) and an increased risk of developing cancer, as well as a correlation between low blood sugar as a hindrance to cancer growth.[33]

- The prognosis of cancer appears to be positively associated with easily available glucose load of the diet.[34] In fact, elevated blood sugar is a predictor of poor survival of cancer patients.[35]

- A multicenter study of 2,500 women showed a direct association between breast cancer risk and higher levels of glycemic index (rate of blood sugar elevation) and glycemic load (average of total daily glucose). The association was even stronger in post-menopausal women.[36]

- Studies at the Longevity Institute of the University of Southern California showed that fasting during chemotherapy slowed the growth of cancer cells faster than either chemotherapy or fasting alone.[37]

- In rats, lowering the carbohydrate content of the diet from 60% energy to 40% energy was sufficient to decrease the rate of tumor growth from 18% to 13% per week.[38] In another study involving mice that normally have a 70-80% chance of developing breast cancer over their lifetime due to genetic mutations, they stayed tumor-free at 1 year of age when their calories from complex carbohydrates were limited to 15%, while almost half of those on a 55% carbohydrate diet developed tumors.[39]

This leads to the natural question: What would be the result if cancer cells could not get easy access to high levels of glucose outside? The logical conclusion is that they may die or not multiply, or we might expect, at the very least, that they would slow down multiplication in a low glucose environment.

# The correlation between glucose and cancer cell multiplication

The markedly increased consumption of glucose for the maintenance, multiplication, movement, and metastasis of cancer cells is established beyond doubt.[40]

In 1885, Ernst Freud found association of elevated blood sugar in 70 out of 70 cancer patients. Physiologist A. Braunstein observed in 1921 that in those diabetic patients who developed cancer, glucose secretion in the urine disappeared. He also showed a much higher consumption of glucose by cancer cells grown in a culture, compared to muscle and liver cells. In 1927 Otto Warburg described that most cancer cells used glucose almost exclusively for their energy production and, unlike normal cells, could extract enough energy from glucose even if oxygen supply was limited. Equally important is the finding in the 1950s by the American physiologist Harry Eagle that cancer cells consume enormous amounts of amino acids compared to normal cells, to manufacture materials needed for new cell formation.

Cancer cells typically have glucose usage up to 200 times higher than normal cells, even if oxygen is plentiful. Therefore, consistently high levels of glucose in the blood, even when the level is not high enough to be in the diabetic range, can provide the energy source for cancer cells to multiply faster than the immune surveillance can destroy them.

When activated for a long time, a subset of cancer cells exhibits the tendency for uncontrolled multiplication even after glucose levels are normalized.[41] This ability occurs because cancer cells often reacquire the characteristics of stem cells with increased survival, migration, and invasion capabilities.[42] In addition, the greater availability of glucose appears to strengthen the resolve of cancer cells to resist self-destruction signals.[43]

In addition, cancer cells release signaling molecules that instruct the liver to produce more glucose molecules from lactate. When lactate molecules reach the liver along with the signaling molecules, the result is more fuel that the cancer cells can then use. In fact, cancer cells can instruct the liver to produce glucose from certain amino acids if no glucose is available from carbohydrate.[44]

## CURIOUS TIDBITS

Patients with cancer often suffer from progressive loss of fat and lean body mass—cancer *cachexia*. This is not caused by nutritional demands, as one does not see a corresponding growth of cancer. Signaling molecules released by cancer cells have been suspected, but why? During prolonged fasting, the body starts degrading proteins, releasing amino acids that could be used to produce glucose in the liver. I suggest that cancer cells have hijacked this normal body process to increase the availability of glucose for their own benefit. Glycerol released during breakdown of fat molecules could also be converted to glucose by the liver.

# What is glucose and how can I avoid it?

You may be wondering what glucose is and what foods that contain it you should avoid. The confusion is that many foods break down into glucose, but there are differences among them, as follows:

- Complex carbohydrates in grains—such as wheat, rice, and corn—and grain-flour products—such as used to make bread, pizza, and pastas—all break down in the small intestine first to *maltose*, and then to the most basic form of sugar, *glucose*.

- Dairy products like milk and cheese have a form of sugar called *lactose*, which is further broken down into *galactose* and *glucose*.

- Fruits also contain a natural sugar, *sucrose*, which is broken down into *fructose* and *glucose*.

You do not need to avoid all of these. The single biggest culprit in putting glucose into your body is complex carbohydrate, specifically from grain products. Grains such as wheat, oats, barley, rye, corn, and rice produce the largest amount of food-associated glucose upon diges- tion. Fruits and dairy produce glucose, but, in a typical American diet, they produce less than grain-based foods. Glucose from fruits and dairy is also released in the intestine at a slower pace.

The body needs some carbohydrates (aka, "carbs"), but the question is, how much? It de- pends to some extent on your age and level of activity.

- Carbs break down into glucose, so the more bread, pasta, and rice you eat, the more you fill your body with glucose.

- Most people consume far more complex carbohydrates than their body can im- mediately use or store.

- Almost all of the excess glucose in your body comes from grain products, making them the most prolific cause of high blood sugar. Eating "whole grain" products does nothing to mitigate the excess glucose that carbs generate in your body.

Unfortunately, food manufacturers are constantly enticing the general population to consume more and more unhealthy, high-carbohydrate grain-based foods: bagels, baguettes, breadsticks, buns, croissants, pretzels, and rolls; challah, chapatti, focaccia, injera, lavash, naan, paratha, pita, pizza, tortilla; bhatura, frybread, puri and sopapilla; biscuits, cakes, crackers, cup- cakes, doughnuts, muffins, and pastries; mantou, pot stickers, dumplings, noodles and other pastas; crepes, pan, pancakes, pandesal, pies, and other food products prepared with grain flours using ethnic cuisines and regional flavors. These all sound so good, don't they? But eating them produces vast amounts of glucose that feeds your cancer cells.

# The difference between maltose, lactose, and sucrose

Many people are confused about whether they are ingesting glucose when they eat fruits, dairy products, or the carbohydrates in grains and grain-flour products. The confusion probably arises because each of these *is* digested into glucose, but at different rates.

- Carbohydrates, found in products made with any type of grain—wheat, oats, barley, rye, rice, corn, and others—break down first into *maltose*. This then is further broken down into 2 molecules of glucose. Both glucose molecules are absorbed quickly into the bloodstream, which is why these carbohydrates boost blood sugar the fastest.

- Fruits, berries, beets, sugar cane, and other products that contain *sucrose* break down into equal parts of glucose and *fructose*. Both are absorbed as they're released in the intestine. But while the glucose part adds to your blood sugar level almost immediately, the fructose part is absorbed only half as fast. Fructose itself must be further processed into glucose before it can elevate your blood sugar level. This means eating a piece of fruit doesn't add the same amount of glucose to your bloodstream as quickly as eating an equal amount of carbohydrate in bread, pizza, or rice.

- Milk sugar, *lactose*, is similar in that it first breaks down into 1 molecule of *galactose* and 1 molecule of glucose. Again, the glucose part is absorbed quickly into the bloodstream, but the galactose must be further processed by the liver and converted to glucose before it can elevate your blood sugar.

The medical profession has done a poor job of educating people on the important differences between these types of foods in how quickly they put glucose into your bloodstream. For example, many people eat muffins, cakes, and pastries made with reduced amounts of sugar (sucrose), believing that they can now consume more of them, without realizing that they are actually consuming more sugar (glucose) from the flour used in the pastry. Eating a piece of fruit for breakfast or as a dessert does not deliver the same immediate glucose impact to your blood as eating a grain-based product such as toast, muffins, cake, or pie; the fruit is effectively healthier for you.

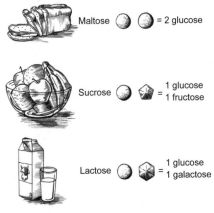

Maltose 〇 〇 = 2 glucose

Sucrose 〇 ⬠ = 1 glucose
1 fructose

Lactose 〇 ⬡ = 1 glucose
1 galactose

Three types of natural sugars: maltose, sucrose, and lactose. Each is composed of a different combination of molecules of sugar. Their different molecular structures mean they break down into glucose at different rates in the body.

# Glucose from carbohydrates is not an essential nutrient you need

The body uses more than 100 different nutrients for human metabolic activities. Some nutrients, however, simply cannot be manufactured internally and so we must consume them in our foods. These are called the essential nutrients, because you must find a way to consume them. These include amino acids, fatty acids, and other essential nutrients such as vitamins and minerals. For example, out of 20 amino acids used by the body, 9 have to be consumed because they can't be manufactured in the body. Similarly, there are essential fatty acids humans must obtain from foods.

However, glucose is not an essential nutrient for humans. It is one of those that can be manufactured inside the body using multiple raw materials. For example, amino acids from plants, nuts, seeds, meat and dairy, lactate (a by-product of incomplete glucose breakdown), oxalate (a product of complete glucose breakdown), and glycerol from each molecule of fat—all these can be used to manufacture glucose in the liver, if and when necessary.

By keeping your blood glucose level at the lowest possible level, which can be done by avoiding the consumption of grains and grain-flour products, you can severely limit the cancer cell's access to glucose, and curtail its further growth and metastasis. The main point is this can be accomplished by avoiding the consumption of grain-based complex carbohydrates, without compromising your intake of needed nutrients.

# The vast amount of glucose in complex carbohydrates

To truly understand the extent of glucose in grain-based complex carbohydrates, it helps to know what complex carbohydrate molecules are.

First, a bond is created between a carbon atom of one glucose molecule and carbon atom of another glucose molecule. Then this process is repeated. For example, starch (a form of complex carbohydrate) is composed of long strings of glucose with branches that also have long strings of glucose. Thousands of glucose molecules can bond together in these long strings. The process is something like the way polycarbonate solid plastic is made by combining carbonate units together. When you bond carbonate units to each other, they get stronger and can be molded into many shapes such as tubes, rods, and sheets, each with different properties of rigidity and heat tolerance.

The properties of starch can be altered by varying how the glucose molecules branch off from the main chain. Wheat, corn, and rice products are effectively large chains of glucose molecules that are neatly folded and tightly compressed to form starches of different solubility, clarity, and responsiveness to chemical and physical conditions. These starches and flours can be used to make numerous dishes, which you may eagerly consume. Then your body breaks down those starches to simpler chains of molecules that end up as glucose molecules, which feed your cancer cells.

# Nature did not intend for humans to consume so much carbohydrate-based glucose

To further reinforce what I have said about carbohydrates, note that muscles (which are the largest user of glucose in the body) can produce energy in two ways.

The first is by converting glucose into ATP in the process called *glycolysis*. This is done outside the cell's mitochondria. Muscle cells do this for about the first 10 seconds of extreme activity.

The second is by burning glucose or fatty acids inside the mitochondria, a process that requires oxygen. When more energy is needed after those first 10 seconds, muscle cells will send out glucose transporters to pick up glucose waiting outside the cell membrane and bring it in. But as your body also has fatty acids in the bloodstream and a large storage of triglycerides in your fat cells, muscle cells will switch to burning fatty acids rather than glucose inside the mitochondria. (If you are wondering why muscle cells switch to burning fatty acids when glucose is still available, let me suggest the following. With fat cells being full, the blood fatty acid level stays high. Those fatty acids can enter muscle cells more easily than glucose, because muscle cell membranes are also made of fatty acids and cholesterol. In addition, adiponectin, a hormone released from fat cells, actively promotes such fatty acid burning. Finally, glucose, being water-soluble, has an outlet from the body through the kidney, unlike fatty acids that have no exit and must be used inside.)

Given that humans are built to store only a small amount (120 grams) of glucose in the liver, this suggests that nature never intended humans to use glucose as our primary method of fueling our muscle cells. Glucose is used for the initial construction of cells (because if no mitochondria yet exists, it is not possible for the cell to burn fatty acids). Glucose is also the primary fuel for nerve cells, including brain cells.

But when it comes to muscles, glucose is simply a "starter" in muscle fibers, used to create a metabolite called *oxaloacetate* that is a kindling agent for energy production from fatty acids inside the mitochondria.

This means that if you stop consuming grains, substantially reducing the amount of glucose produced in the digestive process, your body will still survive by burning fatty acids produced from the foods you consume or from the stored fat in your fat cells. Your liver will automatically produce enough glucose from other nutrients in your food to fuel your nerve cells. Meanwhile, the remaining paucity of glucose in your body gives you your best chance of starving cancer cells, which need glucose to multiply and form new cells. As stated earlier, without glucose cancer cells can't survive, even if your immune system is weak as a result of your treatment.

# The chemistry of cells burning glucose

Glucose is used extensively by cells in the human body because of the ease with which the energy unit ATP can be generated outside the cell's mitochondria. As mentioned, muscle cells depend on glycolysis, the process of breaking glucose down, for about the first 10 seconds of activity. The advantage of this mechanism of energy production is the speed and reliability of producing ATP. The drawback is that not all the extractable energy contained in a molecule of glucose can be extracted by this mechanism. This means that you cannot exert the maximum power that your muscles are capable of, or prolong the activity for a great length of time. To generate extra power, muscles must switch to creating ATP within the mitochondria.

When there is both insulin and glucose outside, insulin tells muscle cells to allow glucose transporters to pick up glucose molecules and bring them inside. But if fatty acids are also present, they will enter the cell without help from insulin. This means that any glucose waiting outside the cell is not needed for energy production, and will remain in the bloodstream. This switch to burning fatty acids is thereby the cause of high blood sugar and Type 2 diabetes.

This may be the reason why nature instituted glycolysis, a reliable and readily available source of ATP, to meet the energy demand of newly forming cells. After all, one needs enough power to generate the mitochondria, which can make up nearly 25% of the total volume of a typical cell, plus energy to create the cell's infrastructure needed for construction, transportation, command and control centers, communications, protection, and waste disposal. It makes sense that nature made glucose the primary energy source for the construction of the basic living cell, a very reliable source for meeting immediate energy needs.

But when it comes to prolonged muscle power, nature arranged cells to use fatty acids to create ATP. When needed, fatty acids, made from excess glucose and stored as fat, can be re-converted to fatty acids to be used to produce energy. Fatty acids cannot be converted back to glucose, no matter how low blood sugar gets.

If glucose were meant to be the primary fuel for energy production in the body, nature would certainly have made provisions for us to have a larger storage capacity than approximately 24 teaspoons at a time of glucose, in the form of glycogen, in the liver. Compare that to our ability to store many, many pounds of fat, with each pound of fat containing approximately 3500 calories, far more than what an adult typically uses on a daily basis.

# Does eating whole grains or gluten-free grains avoid glucose?

All carbohydrates break down into glucose that feeds your cancer cells. It doesn't matter whether the item is whole grain, multi-grain, gluten-free, or refined in any way. Be aware that products made from whole grains contain the same glucose molecules as those made from any other grain. Don't be persuaded by secondary advertising claims such as "no cholesterol," "gluten free," "fortified with vitamins and minerals," and "no high-fructose corn syrup" because such claims do not change the basic composition of these products; they are still foods that will elevate your blood sugar and feed your cancer cells.

When you pick up two pieces of bread, a bun, or a roll to make a sandwich, you are holding long chains of glucose molecules baked to stay firm so you can grasp them. When you flatten dough to make pizza or flat bread, you are shaping glucose molecules into sheets. When you cook noodles and pasta, you are cooking glucose molecules shaped into strings, strips, tubes, shells, or wings. When you make a waffle on a waffle iron or a pancake on a griddle, you are pouring glucose molecules in a batter to make specific formations. The cookie you hold is a piece of glucose sculpture. The mound of rice on your bowl or plate is a heap of glucose.

You would probably never consume an entire bowl of plain sucrose (sugar). Yet this is what you are basically eating when the bowl contains breakfast cereal made from whole grains: essentially, camouflaged glucose molecules. When you eat complex carbohydrate products like a sandwich or pasta, you seldom think that you are eating glucose. When you dip vegetables, fish, shrimp, or meat in a batter of grain flour you do not realize you are coating them with glucose. But this is effectively what you are doing—preparing and eating food that becomes glucose in your blood.

# How much glucose is actually in carbohydrates?

Check the comparisons below to see the equivalent amount of sugar you are eating in your ordinary foods.

Remember this: each 4 grams of carbohydrates you eat is about 1 teaspoon of sugar, and that is equal to millions of glucose molecules.

| Food item | Grams of carbs | Actual Sugar Content (teaspoons) |
| --- | --- | --- |
| Bread, 2 slices | 24 | 6 |
| Breakfast cereal, 1 cup | 30 | 7 ½ |
| 12" sandwich roll (like a sub or hoagie), 1 roll | 36 | 9 |
| Pizza, 1 slice | 40 | 10 |
| Pasta, 2 ounces | 40 | 10 |
| Rice, 1 cup | 48 | 12 |
| Bagel, 1 | 48 | 12 |

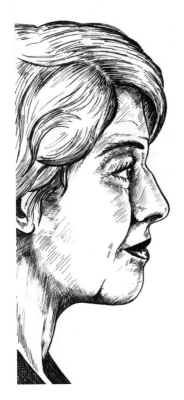

Nature did not intend grain for human consumption. Otherwise, we would have had beaks similar to that of birds. In addition, chaff is not digestible by humans. It is mechanized farming, milling, and refining that have made it easier for humans to consume enormous amounts of glucose strung together as complex carbohydrate in grains, an ideal fuel and raw material for construction of cancer cells.

# Reducing your consumption of grains is especially vital for diabetics with cancer

If you are a diabetic or prediabetic with cancer, you may incur a double threat.

First, as you learned earlier, the consumption of grains produces voluminous amounts of glucose that, unless you are active, are probably more than your energy needs at any given time. Your liver can store only 120 grams of glucose, and the rest of that glucose enters your bloodstream. If you have been active, some of that glucose may go to restore glycogen in your muscles; but if you have been sedentary, most of the excess glucose ends up in the liver to be converted to triglycerides for storage in your fat cells. The problem is, when your fat cells are full, limited by the storage capacity you inherited, and the number of fat stem cells your body manufactured based on maternal nutrition when you were in the womb, it causes the excess glucose to remain in your bloodstream—available to feed your cancer cells.

Secondly, as soon as you have glucose in your bloodstream, it triggers your brain to instruct your pancreas to begin producing insulin, the hormone that tells cells to allow the glucose in. Herein lies the double threat. As you learned earlier, insulin actually helps cancer cells multiply. Recall that insulin helps induce the formation of enzymes needed for glycolysis, the process of extracting ATP from glucose molecules, the fuel that cancer cells thrive on. In addition to helping cancer cells produce needed energy, insulin also inhibits cellular "stickiness," so cancer cells get more freedom to move out of their tumor mass, i.e., to metastasize.

The statistics about cancer among people with diabetes support this conclusion. People with fasting blood glucose levels exceeding 100 milligrams per deciliter, especially after age 50, have a higher risk of death from cancer—on average, six years earlier than a person without high blood sugar. Furthermore, as fasting blood sugar increases, so does the risk of cancer.[45] In scientific terms, this is called *a dose response*, indicating a higher expected occurrence of an event when the causative factor is stronger.

In a nutshell, if you can keep your blood sugar low, and avoid having to inject insulin or taking medications that cause the release of insulin in your body, you will be depriving cancer cells of their needed fuel for growth, while limiting the critical growth promoter in the form of insulin.

# Will I lack energy if I give up the carbohydrates in grains?

As mentioned earlier, food energy enters the body as glucose, amino acid, or fatty acid. So you may think that, based on the way you have been eating all your life, you may not have energy to function well if you completely give up grain and grain-based foods. However, I suggest that, while starving cancer cells by limiting grains and grain-flour products, you can still feel energetic by eating more of proteins and fat.

Every cell in the body is capable of using glucose as a fuel to produce ATP (adenosine triphosphate). In a normal cell, after the initial breakdown of a glucose molecule (the process known as *glycolysis*), the intermediate product formed is further metabolized inside the mitochondria, the cell's powerhouse, to extract the maximum amount of energy from each glucose molecule. This process requires a steady supply of oxygen.

But whenever your body is lacking glucose, such as between meals or during heavy exercise, normal cells will burn small fatty acid compounds produced by the liver from larger fatty acid molecules released from your fat cells, as an alternate fuel in the mitochondria—instead of glucose. In other words, your body is perfectly capable of surviving and having plenty of energy without consuming grains to produce glucose.

However, you need to watch out for overconsuming protein and fat in an attempt to avoid grain and grain-flour products. If you do that, the muscles could switch to burning fatty acids, as mentioned above. Amino acids absorbed into the body after proteins are digested can be converted into glucose by your liver. In other words, if your total energy intake is more than what you can utilize before your next meal, you may still have a higher blood sugar level than if your total energy intake is lower.

In comparison, cancer cells cannot live without glucose, their main source of energy. Recall that cancer cells are not capable of producing energy from fatty acids, because they do not have functioning mitochondria where this alternate fuel is used. So avoiding the consumption of grains can starve cancer cells, without affecting your energy needs. But you have to also pay attention to your total energy intake.

# Which is more important: Treating your diabetes or treating your cancer?

If you have diabetes and control it by injecting insulin or taking medications that help your pancreas produce more insulin, you might be feeling that you are caught between needing to control your diabetes versus taking steps to eliminate your cancer.

There is only one answer to this quandary. Stopping your cancer is most important. And in the process of doing that, it is highly likely that you will also end up gaining control of your high blood sugar. Check with your diabetes care provider as to the best way to reduce and potentially stop taking insulin or medications that cause release of insulin from your pancreas.

My suggestion is based on the following reasoning. In the body, the glucose utilization system consists of two critical steps: the transfer of glucose from the intestine into the blood, and the entry of glucose into the cell. The second part is beyond your control; you cannot prevent it. But the first part is not. You can prevent a major portion of glucose from being in your intestines—by not consuming grains!

Therefore, if you have cancer, your goal should be to reduce your intake of glucose-producing grains to as close to zero as possible. This does not mean you will not have any energy. Remember that your muscle cells can derive energy from burning the fatty acids stored in your fat cells, and your liver can produce glucose for your brain cells by combining amino acids from the foods you eat other than carbohydrates.

# How much carbohydrate does your body need?

In a healthy person, glucose occupies a central position in metabolic activities. A typical cell in the body has the capacity to make about 30,000 different proteins. Glucose can not only provide energy needed for activities but can also be a precursor for the production of amino acids, fatty acids, and other products. As a result, we might say that a healthy body benefits from some carbohydrates—but how much? It depends on age and level of activity.

The main use of glucose is as a fuel. During infancy and childhood, our carbohydrate needs are very high relative to our body size because we are rapidly growing cells in almost every organ. A developing infant's body requires an abundance of energy to duplicate cells and internal structures, which take their instructions from growth hormone released from the pituitary gland. Cell division is like splitting a house into two, with each half being transformed into a new house with its own walls, appliances, plumbing, wiring, waste disposal, and heating. Those houses then split in two yet again, as the cell division process continues.

As we approach adulthood, and we continue to be healthy, we need less glucose for two reasons. First, our cells multiply more slowly because new cells are mostly formed to replace dead cells within organs, rather than to build new structures. As a result, there is reduced glucose need for cell division. As we age, there is also usually a reduction in muscle mass, so there are fewer cells where glucose can be stored as muscle glycogen. Reduced muscle mass also means reduced energy needs.

# Grains, Glucose, and Cancer

Total global grain production increased from 0.8 billion metric tons in 1961 to 2.8 billion metric tons in 2014, while the world population increased from 3 billion to 7 billion. Nearly every industrialized country in the world today utilizes vast quantities of grains—wheat, oats, barley, corn, rice, and others—and this parallels the increasing incidence of lifestyle-related conditions such as obesity, diabetes, and cancer. The fact is, the consumption of grains and grain-based food products is not necessary for human well-being.

This is the story of grains in relation to cancer—and why you want to reduce your consumption of them to as close to zero as possible.

---

The ancestors of modern humans appeared on earth about 50,000 years ago. Cultivation of plants started only after 40,000 years of human existence. This means that humans survived without consuming significant amounts of grain and grain products for a majority of human history. The domestication and cultivation of rice and grains like wheat and rye dates back to only about 13,000 to 10,000 BCE. This was a major lifestyle change; human patterns of hunting and gathering changed to farming crops and raising domesticated animal-based foods.

Humans were always equipped to break down complex carbohydrates, as shown by the presence in the intestine of *amylase*, the enzyme that digests complex carbohydrates. But it's likely that early humans obtained complex carbohydrates and carbohydrate-associated nutrients from vegetables that required chewing, such as yam, cassava, potato, and taro. Even today, humans do live in regions of the world where grain farming is not possible or where grains are not available on a regular basis. The lack of human physiology to remove the chaff from a grain kernel before consumption, as is the case with birds having a beak, is indicative of the fact that grains were not necessary for human survival.

It was not until several millennia ago that carbohydrate from grains became a staple of the human diet. The ancient Egyptians learned to farm wheat in the fertile Nile Valley. Asian cultures farmed rice. In the middle ages, many cultures survived on porridge, rice, or potatoes, depending on which crops grew in their region. In the late 19th century, industrialized roller mills were invented, making it easier to refine grains into flour, which could then be used to make other products. Because of this, grains have become the major source of carbohydrate in human diets in most populated areas of the world. In many countries, grains provide 50% or more of the energy in their diets.

Today, modern agricultural practices allow us to cultivate hybridized, drought-resistant crops using irrigation, fertilizer, and machinery to produce an abundance of grains to feed humanity. The top three crops produced in the world are rice, maize (corn), and wheat. Each is cultivated at a level of 600 to 800 million metric tons per year in order to feed billions of people around the globe and to provide nutrition for the animals we eat.

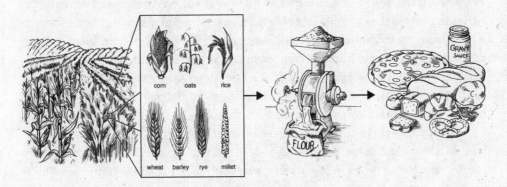

In general, grains are easy to transport, fast to cook, easy to chew, and easily digested and absorbed (except by people with celiac disease or grain allergies). Milling grains to create flour makes them easy to store without refrigeration. Refining produces starches and flours with qualities that chefs can exploit to create a multitude of dishes and products. For example, wheat can be refined into flour with a high protein content to make crusty or chewy breads, or low protein content suitable for cakes, cookies, and piecrusts. Wheat flour is also used to thicken gravy and sauces. The variety of edible products that can be made with the carbohydrate from grains is never-ending, and these food items throughout the world tempt us.

## Grains flood you with glucose

Grains are complex carbohydrates, meaning they are long chains of glucose. In digestion, they are broken down first into molecules of maltose, which is then further digested into glucose. Each molecule of maltose produces two molecules of glucose, as opposed to fruit sugar (sucrose), which breaks down into one molecule of fructose and one molecule of glucose, and milk sugar (lactose), which breaks down into one molecule of galactose and one molecule of glucose. In other words, grains produce twice as much as glucose as fruit and milk sugars.

When you eat bread, pita, naan, pizza, cakes, muffins, pies, chips, pretzels, taco shells, tortillas, rice, corn, and hundreds of other products made with grain flours, you are effectively eating millions of molecules of glucose. Every cell keeps some glucose stored in the form of glycogen that is essentially a complex carbohydrate similar to starch. The liver also stores glycogen, but only 120 grams at any given time, to be released back into the blood to maintain circulating blood sugar level. When glycogen stores are filled, the excess absorbed glucose is stored as fat, so the energy can be used at a later time. In other words, consuming grains basically forces your body to store excess glucose in your fat cells. This situation is the perfect setup for Type 2 diabetes and cancer, which I will discuss shortly.

## Why we are attracted to carbohydrates

While we do not need grains, it is natural that the sweetness of glucose from carbohydrates appeals to the human sense of taste. Our experience with sweet taste starts as a baby when we consume lactose (milk sugar) as well as sucrose from fruits and berries. Both galactose and fructose, components of lactose and sucrose respectively, can eventually be converted into glucose by the liver. When any of these sugars come into contact with the sweet-sensing taste buds in the mouth, signals are sent to the brain, producing the sensation of sweetness.

When you begin to eat a meal, the result is elevated blood sugar, which reassures the brain that glucose has been received as expected, a state of starvation has been averted, and fuel in the form of glucose is available for immediate or future use. This is especially important for neurons in the brain because they preferentially use glucose to produce energy needed for metabolic activities. The sensation of sweetness is the reward for fulfilling the need.

Through repetition of this experience, when any type of sugar stimulates the sweet-sensing taste buds, it produces a pleasing response because your brain has a "learned experience" of satisfaction based on nutritive value. Over time, the body associates the sweet taste with the imminent arrival of glucose in the blood. This is similar to you receiving a paycheck. From experience, you know what it represents—money soon to be available in your bank account.

## The benefits of carbohydrate

Humans need glucose as fuel for our cells and our primary source of glucose is carbohydrates, found in a wide variety of foods, including vegetables, grains, and dairy.

Carbohydrate in the form of dissolved glucose is always present in the blood and in the fluid around cells. The normal blood glucose concentration in a person who has not eaten a meal within the past three to four hours is 90 milligrams/deciliter (mg/dl). In a normal person, about an hour after a meal containing a large amount of carbohydrates—such as bread, pasta, rice, or corn—the blood glucose level will seldom rise above 140 mg/dl because most of the glucose enters into the cells of the body, where it is used for energy. Glucose also remains in the fluid around cells, usually in the range of 75 to 95 mg/dl, though it can fluctuate in the short term between 20 and 1500 mg/dl without any harmful consequences. If the blood glucose level falls below one-half of normal, people usually experience a loss of mental functions—confusion, forgetfulness, and lack of analytic capabilities.

Carbohydrates in the form of fructose and galactose perform specialized functions in cell membranes. For example, these sugars combine with protein or fat molecules that dangle outside cell walls and repel charged particles because of their negative charge. These combined structures attach themselves to carbohydrates protruding from other cells to maintain the cohesion of cells within an organ.

These combined structures also act as receptors for binding hormones in cells and participate in our immune defense mechanisms by attacking bacteria in the blood, saliva, and tears. The identification of your blood type as A, B, AB, or O is based on the presence of these structures on the red cell membrane. In addition, a special carbohydrate molecule is used in the construction of genes that reside inside the control center of each cell (the nucleus), and a variation of that molecule is used to manufacture the messenger that carries instructions from genes to workers in the cell.

But humans can also get our cellular fuel from fatty acids, produced from the fats we consume, as well as from triglycerides that the liver produces from excess glucose. In climates that do not allow people to grow grains or have easy access to vegetables, the liver can produce glucose from amino acids derived from proteins. For example, the indigenous Inuit people of Northern Canada and Alaska can live for long periods of time on a diet that provides approximately 50% of their calories from fat. Their livers produce glucose from the amino acids in meat. In addition, they burn extensive amounts of acetyl-coenzyme A (acetyl-CoA), derived from fat, as fuel in their cells. Thus, nature has protected the Inuit, who have little carbohydrate available to them in their diet.

## Why you don't need carbohydrates from grains

Most importantly, while we need carbohydrates, we do not need them in the volume that today's diets of three meals per day, plus snacks, often provide. And the main culprit in today's diets is carbohydrate from grains.

Diabetes specialists justify the intake of grain by saying that glucose is an important nutrient. However, as mentioned, the body can only store in reserve a small amount (120 grams) of glucose in the liver. Glucose molecules that cells don't take inside within four hours of absorption into the blood are converted to fatty acids for long-term storage in your fat cells, to be used for energy production as needed. (Note: If you keep eating every four hours, you may seldom dip into your fat storage, and that is why you gain weight.) And given that the body also makes glucose from foods we eat other than grain-based carbohydrates, the chances are that you are frequently overloading your body's capacity to utilize glucose. It does not matter the type of food the body acquires the glucose from—120 grams are 120 grams! If you consume a heavy meal with a sandwich, meat, chips, and a dessert, you may be over the threshold of what the body can typically use over four hours.

As the table below shows, grains contain far more carbohydrate than any vegetable. Remember: each 4 grams of carbohydrate is equal to 1 teaspoon of sugar.

## Table 1. Comparison of carbs in grains vs. vegetables

| Food item | Grams of carbs |
|---|---|
| Bread, 2 slices | 24 |
| Breakfast cereal, 1 cup | 30 |
| 12" sandwich roll (like a sub or hoagie), 1 roll | 36 |
| Pizza, 1 slice | 40 |
| Pasta, 2 ounces | 40 |
| Rice, 1 cup | 48 |
| Bagel, 1 | 48 |
| Alfalfa sprouts, raw, 100g | 0.4 |
| Artichoke Jerusalem, boiled, 100g | 10.6 |
| Asparagus, boiled, 100g | 4 |
| Bamboo shoots, canned, 100g | 0.7 |
| Beansprouts, mung, raw, 100g | 4 |
| Beetroot, boiled, 100g | 9.5 |
| Broccoli, green, boiled, 100g | 1.3 |
| Broccoli, purple, boiled, 100g | 1.3 |
| Brussels Sprouts, boiled, 100g | 3.1 |
| Cabbage, spring, boiled, 100g | 0.6 |
| Cabbage, Chinese, raw, 100g | 1.4 |
| Cabbage, red, raw, 100g | 3.7 |
| Cabbage, Savoy, raw, 100g | 3.9 |
| Cabbage, white, raw, 100g | 5 |
| Capsicum Pepper, green, raw 100g | 2.6 |
| Capsicum Pepper, red, raw 100g | 6.4 |
| Carrots, young, raw, 100g | 6 |
| Cauliflower, boiled, 100g | 2.3 |
| Celery, raw, 100g | 0.9 |
| Corn, baby sweetcorn, boiled, 100g | 2.7 |
| Corn kernels, canned, 100g | 2.7 |
| Corn-on-cob, boiled, plain, 100g | 11.6 |
| Curly Kale, raw, 100g | 1.4 |
| Cucumber, unpeeled, raw 100g | 1.5 |

| Food item | Grams of carbs |
| --- | --- |
| Eggplant, raw, 100g | 2.2 |
| Endive (Escarole), 100g | 2.8 |
| Fennel, raw, 100g | 1.8 |
| Garlic, fresh, raw, 100g | 33 |
| Leeks, raw, 100g | 2.9 |
| Lettuce, cos, romaine, raw, 100g | 1.7 |
| Lettuce, Iceberg, raw, 100g | 1.9 |
| Mushrooms, common, raw, 100g | 3.4 |
| Potatoes, new, boiled, 100g | 18 |
| Onions, raw, 100g | 7.9 |
| Parsnip, raw, 100g | 12.5 |
| Peas, frozen, raw, 100g | 9.3 |
| Peas, fresh, raw, 100g | 11.3 |
| Radish, red, raw, 100g | 2 |
| Spinach, raw, 100g | 1.6 |
| Squash, butternut, baked, 100g | 7.4 |
| Squash, spaghetti, baked, 100g | 1.8 |
| Zucchini, raw, 100g | 1.8 |
| Sweet potato, baked, 100g | 28 |
| Tomatoes, canned, & liquid, 100g | 3 |
| Tomatoes, cherry, raw, 100g | 3 |
| Yam, baked, 100g | 37.5 |

## You don't need grains for their other nutrients

Another claim is that other nutrients associated with grains are also important. But as Table 2 shows, you can get nearly all the grain-associated nutrients from vegetables, nuts, fruits, and mushrooms. Use of spices and herbs will give you even more opportunities to get needed nutrients without having to consume the voluminous amount of glucose, of which thousands of molecules are present in each molecule of complex carbohydrate and constitute the bulk of a grain kernel. Moreover, grains contain only a fraction of over 100 nutrients the body uses on a daily basis. In other words, there is no health benefit from eating grains, even if you don't consume animal products.

**Table 2.** Comparison of nutrients from various grains vs. lentils, brazil nuts, raisins, and mushrooms

| 100g portion | Wheat | Brown Rice | Corn | Lentils | Brazil nuts | Raisins | Mushrooms |
|---|---|---|---|---|---|---|---|
| Fiber (g) | 12.2 | 3.5 | 7.3 | 10.7 | 7.5 | 3.7 | — |
| Calcium (mg) | 29 | 23 | 7 | 56 | 160 | 50 | 18 |
| Iron (mg) | 3.2 | 1.4 | 2.7 | 6.5 | 2.4 | 1.9 | 0.4 |
| Magnesium(mg) | 126 | 143 | 127 | 47 | 376 | 32 | 9 |
| Phosphorus(mg) | 288 | 333 | 210 | 281 | 725 | 24 | 120 |
| Potassium(mg) | 363 | 223 | 287 | 677 | 659 | 749 | 448 |
| Sodium (mg) | 2 | 7 | 35 | 6 | 3 | 11 | 6 |
| Zinc (mg) | 2.6 | 2.0 | 2.2 | 3.3 | 4.0 | 0.2 | 1.1 |
| Copper (mg) | 0.4 | | 0.3 | — | — | — | 0.5 |
| Manganese(mg) | 3.9 | 3.7 | 0.4 | — | — | 0.3 | — |
| Selenium (mg) | 70.7 | — | 15.5 | — | 1917 (ug) | | 26 (ug) |
| Thiamin (mg) | 0.4 | 0.4 | 0.3 | 0.8 | 0.6 | 0.1 | 0.1 |
| Riboflavin (mg) | 0.1 | 0.1 | 0.2 | 0.2 | — | 0.1 | 0.5 |
| Niacin (mg) | 5.4 | 5.0 | 3.6 | 2.6 | — | 0.8 | 3.8 |
| Pantothenic acid (mg) | 0.9 | 1.5 | 0.4 | 2.1 | — | 0.1 | 1.5 |
| Vitamin B6 (mg) | 0.3 | 0.5 | 0.6 | 0.5 | — | 0.1 | 0.1 |
| Folate Total (ug) | 38 | 20 | 19 | 479 | 22 | 5 | 25 |

## Have our bodies adapted to high carbohydrate consumption?

Is there any evidence that humans have evolved to accommodate such an excess of carbohydrate in the form of glucose molecules absorbed after a meal containing 50% of energy from grain products?

One theory is that some humans did undergo a genetic mutation that allows us to store excess food intake in our fat cells. The presumption was that this mutation helped our ancient ancestors living in challenging climates or situations to survive during periods of famine. In this theory, the mutation gave them large fat storage capacities, using a larger number of fat cells and/or larger-size fat cells.

The problem with this theory is that no such genes have been identified. In addition, the very presence of lean people, even in regions that have experienced significant famine for many generations, would seem to contradict the theory.

This suggests that human fat storage capacity has not expanded relative to significantly increased consumption of grain-based complex carbohydrates that has happened over the past several centuries. It seems that the shift to grains has occurred too recently to have caused mutations leading to any beneficial adaptations in our genes to accommodate the large amount of grains that most cultures now consume.[46]

## The misleading science about fats pushed us into grains

In the US, one of the major factors behind the enormous expansion of carbohydrates in our diets arose out of a misguided (and highly manipulated) war against fat. In the mid-1980s, a million Americans were dying from heart disease, believed to be caused by low-density lipoprotein (LDL) cholesterol. The National Institutes of Health recommended that all Americans eat less fat and cholesterol to reduce the risk of heart disease.

In response, the food industry promulgated the virtues of "healthy" carbohydrates over fats, suggesting that people need to eat more grains and "whole grains." Americans bought into this science and increased their intake of carbohydrate while reducing their consumption of fat, starting in infancy and continuing through childhood and adulthood.

Carbohydrate intake now accounts for over 50% of the calories in the typical adult diet in the US. Many expert panels encourage the consumption of "whole" grain products, believing in their health benefits just because they contain B vitamins, vitamin E, and fiber normally associated with bran. The medical community further aids this process with pronouncements exalting the virtues of eating the first meal—usually some grain-based cereal, oatmeal, or bread—that gets you ready for the day. They emphasize this directive by warning that those who don't have breakfast are likely to consume a mid-morning snack containing more energy than they would have consumed at breakfast.

The food industry has been happy to exploit this opportunity by marketing easy-to-prepare cereals and many grain-based products for breakfast. The food companies even procure endorsements from medical associations and experts regarding products made with whole grains, the virtues of the vitamins, minerals, and proteins they have added to grain-based products, or the deletion of particles such as gluten from these products. Focusing on these supposed health benefits in their advertising has made it easier for the general population to completely overlook the serious impact that the carbs in these foods have on their blood glucose levels.

This cavalier attitude towards the medically unsound nature of excessive carbohydrate diets has given food manufacturers ammunition to entice the general population to consume more and more grain-based foods: bagels, baguettes, breadsticks, buns, croissants, pretzels, and rolls; challah, chapatti, focaccia, injera, lavash, naan, paratha, pita, pizza, and tortilla; bhatura, frybread, puri, and sopaipilla; biscuits, cakes, crackers, cupcakes, doughnuts, muffins, and pastries; mantou, pot stickers, dumplings, noodles, and other pastas; crepes, pan, pancakes, pandesal, pies, and other food products prepared with grain flours using ethnic cuisines and regional flavors.

These all sound so good, don't they? But eating them may be putting you at risk of high blood sugar and diabetes. In fact, the evidence is clear: the prevalence of Type 2 diabetes in the US increased over 160 percent from 1980 to 2012, along with the increase in obesity and overweight. According to a 2014 analysis of health survey data, individuals born between the years 1966 to 1980 are twice as likely to have diabetes compared to individuals of the same age born between 1946 and 1965.

It is also not surprising that we now see an increasing incidence of weight gain and associated conditions such as Type 2 diabetes in other regions of the world where easily digestible grain-based carbohydrates have become the main staple.

## My theory about why grains cause type 2 diabetes

The medical community has long believed that Type 2 diabetes is caused by insulin resistance, though little is known about how cells develop this "resistance" to a natural hormone produced in the pancreas. Some theorists speculate that something triggers cells to become resistant to insulin, the hormone that facilitates the entry of glucose into cells, but no mechanism has ever been demonstrated.

I suggest that, given the link between the increase in grain consumption, obesity, and Type 2 diabetes, it is grains and the voluminous amount of glucose that they produce that cause high blood sugar, leading to prediabetes and Type 2 diabetes.

Here is how it happens. Following each meal, carbohydrates are digested and converted down to glucose in the intestine. Absorbed into the blood from the intestine, glucose molecules circulate around cells to be picked up. Any glucose in the bloodstream that does not enter cells flows back into the liver, which then uses some of it to produce glycogen. About 120 grams of glycogen are stored in the liver available to release glucose back into the bloodstream to keep blood sugar levels normal between meals.

The problem is that once the liver has made enough glycogen, any additional excess glucose is converted into fatty acids and eventually to triglycerides that are sent to your fat cells for storage. Over time, the consumption of carbohydrates eventually causes many people to fill their fat cells. As mentioned earlier, based on inheritance and the availability of fat stem cells, everyone has a specific fat storage capacity, and when that is filled, those triglycerides simply can no longer fit in. The triglycerides and fatty acids then accumulate in your blood.

What you need to understand, however, is that muscle cells burn fatty acids on a regular basis. Between meals, or when you have exercised heavily, your muscle cells have switched to using fatty acids to create the energy, ATP, that fuels their activities. When you consume grains over time, filling your fat cells and eventually putting fatty acids into your bloodstream, your muscle cells begin burning those fatty acids on a constant basis, rather than glucose. The use of fatty acids for energy production leaves glucose in the blood in excess of what is necessary for basal metabolic needs, even in the fasting stage. The result of this "fatty acid burn switch" is what leads to high blood sugar (prediabetes), as well as Type 2 diabetes and complications associated with this condition.

My theory on this cause of high blood sugar and Type 2 diabetes is far more logical than the theory of insulin resistance, which has, in fact, never been proven. My theory also helps us understand why people with Type 2 diabetes have a higher incidence of cancer than those who do not have the condition.

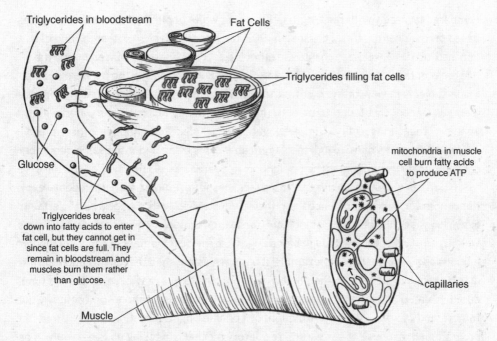

The "fatty acid burn switch" is the cause of high blood sugar and diabetes. The overconsumption of grains fills your fat cells, causing triglycerides that break down into fatty acids to have no place to be stored. Muscles burn those fatty acids rather than glucose.

## The link between grains and cancer

A high correlation seen between individuals who have Type 2 diabetes and those developing cancer leads to the possibility that the consumption of carbohydrates from grains not only is the cause of Type 2 diabetes, but also plays a role in encouraging cancer growth and metastasis.

One proof of this theory can be seen by comparing individuals who get cancer in an environment of excess glucose with those who don't—namely our ancestor hunter-gatherer tribes. For example, cancer has been reported to be very rare among uncivilized hunter-gatherer societies, such as the Native Americans.[47]

What could be the reason for this finding? It could be that they had much more physical activity than we moderns, and plenty of sun exposure resulting in vitamin-D production. They probably also got adequate sleep, and lived life at a reduced stress level. Of course, we cannot dispute that these primitive peoples suffered a much higher rate of infectious diseases compared to modern humans. But perhaps this made it possible for them to develop a robust immune system that may have helped them fight off cancer. And chances are those immune capabilities were codified with gene mutations, which were then passed on to successive generations.

But could the rare occurrence of cancer among the American Indians be due to reduced average length of life compared to the white population? The answer seems to be no, as it has been established that the average longevity of the American Indian compared favorably with the length of life of the white population in the United States, based on the twelfth official census. In 1903, the Imperial Cancer Research Fund of London instituted an investigation into the ethnological distribution of cancer among the native races of the British Colonies. The American Indians residing in the US were excellent study subjects in view of the fact that the government kept a record of each individual member. Cancer was found to be extremely rare among Indians as compared with the whites of the same locality. The investigators concluded that although cancer prevails among all the races of mankind, the American Indians living under the same geographical and climatic conditions as their neighbors appeared nearly immune from the disease.

No matter how we analyze it, the exact reason for hunter-gatherer people experiencing lower cancer incidences is difficult to establish with any degree of certainty. However, we could look for a significant correlation between environmental food cues, weight gain, and obesity with high blood sugar and the development of cancer in modern humans as an explanation. For example, it has been established that environmental stimuli may cause overeating to the point of weight gain. People may overeat due to stimuli directly related to food—taste, availability, or attractive presentation—or it could be due to non-food factors—stress, distraction, or conditioning. Overeating could also be the programmed response of our natural regulatory mechanism telling us to eat more in order to get a much-needed nutrient that is present in only minute quantities in our foods.

However, we know that nature also has compensatory mechanisms that encourage us to reduce our food intake to deal with short-term weight gain so we can maintain stable weight in the long-term.[48] In other words, not everyone who eats in excess from time to time keeps on gaining weight to the point of developing obesity and weight-related complications such as diabetes and cancer.

But another factor could be at play in the lack of cancer development among our hunter-gatherer ancestors. This is the fact that they ate almost no grains. Rather, they derived their energy from foods probably more like what we today call the "paleo diet," consisting of meat, vegetables, fruits, nuts, and roots. They did not eat bread, cakes, pies, pizza, and so many other products made with grains. Their consumption of foods that become glucose in digestion was minimal compared to the amount of carbohydrate that we moderns consume.

The same link to grains that I have theorized as the cause of Type 2 diabetes is what I believe is behind the increased rate of cancer among diabetics as well as an increased risk of cancer among non-diabetics. As stated above, grains digest into voluminous amounts of glucose.

Is there any evidence of this? How might we see that glucose from grains rather than from other carbohydrates could be responsible for cancer formation? The answer becomes obvious given what we know about cancer. In order for a mutated cell to become cancer and multiply, it needs:

- a reliable energy source,
- nutrients for new cell construction as cancer cells multiply, and
- a growth promoter to stimulate cancer cell multiplication.

Eating grains fulfills all three of these requirements. Here's how.

**A reliable energy source:** As the entries in the main part of this book explain, grains produce voluminous amounts of glucose, which is precisely the reliable energy source cancer cells need. Without functional mitochondria, cancer cells rely on glucose to produce the ATP that powers their tasks, especially their ability to multiply. Cancer cells cannot use fatty acids to produce ATP in the mitochondria the way normal cells do, and therefore, to stay alive, they aggressively seek out any glucose in the vicinity of their locale.

**Nutrients for new cell construction:** Cancer cells also release messengers to go outside the cell with instructions to construct new blood vessels and connect them to any available blood vessels in the vicinity. This ensures a steady supply of glucose, which they rob from other cells. For example, the ability of human lung cancer cells to manufacture extra glucose transporters, aggressively absorb glucose molecules, grow indiscriminately and endanger life has been demonstrated.[49] In addition, enhanced expression of genes leading to cancer cell growth and proliferation by the availability of glucose, and reduced expression when they were deprived of glucose has also been demonstrated.[50]

In addition, the more carbohydrate from grains we eat, the more digestion stimulates the production of insulin, which in turn makes you hungry. This is because

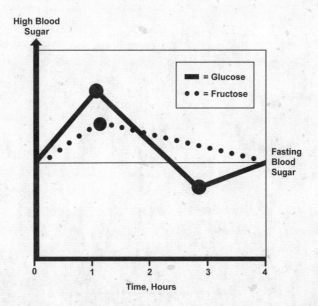

When you eat foods containing grains, your blood sugar skyrockets during the immediate hour following consumption. This causes release of a large amount of insulin from the pancreas that, in turn, results in blood sugar plummeting and even going below fasting level. This now alerts the brain to create the hunger sensation and directs you to eat food containing glucose or sugar. It is likely you will eat more grain-based foods and thus gain weight.

However, when you consume fruit, your blood sugar rises at a slower pace because the fructose takes longer to digest into glucose. Your blood sugar thus descends more slowly in alignment with your insulin level.

ingesting foods that digest into glucose produces a steep elevation of plasma glucose and insulin levels for about an hour after consumption. However, this steep increase is followed by a steep decline. Then 2 to 3 hours after ingesting glucose, plasma glucose levels actually fall below fasting levels for a time, while insulin remains elevated.

With low blood glucose and high insulin, the body begins feeling hungry, craving more glucose.[51] In fact, participants given access to food at this time consumed 500 more calories compared to those who were given fructose that was equal in caloric value and carbohydrate content as that in the glucose load, under the same experimental conditions. In addition, the increase in plasma glucose and insulin was much more gradual in those who consumed fructose. We see this in the typical scenario in most households in the United States. An early morning breakfast based on grain-flour based products such as cereal, toast, bagel, muffin, pancake, croissant, waffle, or a roll leads to the desire to have a mid-morning snack because of the high insulin/low glucose response in the body, as explained above. Almost invariably, what is easily available and what most people resort to eating is another grain-flour product.

Then a lunch consisting of over 50% of the energy coming from grain-flour products such as pasta, sandwich bread, rice, pizza, noodles, etc. leads to the desire to have a mid-afternoon snack based on the same reason as above. Again, what is consumed? Cakes, cupcakes, brownies, cookies, pretzels, etc. and these are also made with grain

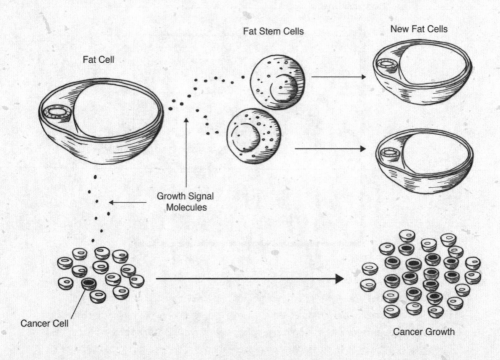

Overeating grains can fill your fat cells and cause growth signal molecules to tell the body to produce more fat cells. However, the same growth signaling molecules may also stimulate cancer cells to multiply. The conclusion: avoid weight gain that might stimulate the release of growth-signaling molecules.

flour. An evening meal could also have over 50% of the energy coming from grain-flour products, followed by a dessert containing grain flour.

As you can see, eating grains leads to a perpetual cycle of high blood sugar and associated high insulin levels, followed by low blood glucose causing hunger and the desire to eat more carbohydrates that increases blood sugar. This circularity prevents the execution of food intake moderation that would have normally happened if our natural regulatory mechanisms of hunger and satiation were allowed to function. The result is increased food intake and weight gain. Worse, the increased food intake itself provides plenty of raw materials available for construction of new cells—normal or cancerous.

*A growth promoter:* This daily overconsumption of grains leads to several results that aid cancer cells. First, gaining weight from overconsumption leads to filling up one's fat cells. Then, as available fat cells are filled to capacity, they release growth-promoting signals to induce the production of more fat cells from available stem cells. The problem is, those same growth-promoting signals also stimulate cancer cells to multiply.

In addition, it has been shown that elevation of blood glucose level after a meal stimulates the secretion of insulin and chronically elevated concentrations of insulin appear to influence cancer growth.[52]

Finally, when fat cells are eventually full, and the body can no longer transform stem cells into more fat cells, there is nowhere for excess glucose to go. As the main portion of the book has stated, this excess glucose is converted into small fatty acid compounds, which muscles switch to burning rather than their normal metabolism of burning glucose. This, in turn, leads to a further elevation of blood sugar, which further feeds cancer cells.

## Avoiding grains is your chance to halt metastasis

I hope I have stated my reasons for limiting the entry of glucose into the body convincingly. The key to surviving cancer is thus to limit the entry of glucose into the body. Even if you have already been diagnosed with cancer, you need to refrain from eating grains to accomplish this. This may effectively limit the growth of those cancer cells, as well as prevent them from spreading to other parts of the body.

Before I explain the strategy to employ to avoid grains, let me clarify one thing—no one can yet stop the random transition of a normal cell into cancer cell. As the beginning of this book informed you, any cell can undergo gene mutation at any time. Unless we learn to stop all mutations forever, we cannot halt the accidental formation of a cancer cell. We need mutations for the survival of the human race, as our evolution requires beneficial mutations that we do not want to prevent from happening. And as noted earlier, most of the currently available therapies, even with early detection, cannot be depended upon to ensure complete eradication of all cancer cells from the body anyway.

Don't get me wrong; I endorse attempts by cancer specialists to discover and offer new treatments that fit a patient's need. However, the limitation I see is that science may not be able to keep up with cancer's trickiness. While a new treatment

## Enjoyment of grains

I t is true that some people enjoy eating whole grain, brown or wild rice, and even white rice. This, in fact, can help them control the quantity consumed by stopping eating when the intensity of enjoyment diminishes.

However, chances are that what you enjoy when you eat grains or food containing grain-flour are actually the vitamins and minerals your nutrient-counting brain has come to associate with that particular carbohydrate, as well as any spices, sugar, salt, oil, or fat added to it. In reality, your enjoyment is based on nutrients other than what is in the complex carbohydrates you eat. You're unlikely to be aware of how bland most grains and grain-flour foods are because you typically eat them topped with butter, jam, jelly, cheese, salt, syrup, seasonings, gravy, sauce, or other condiments. The danger is that if your body identifies an immediate need for a nutrient present in minute quantity in that item, you may feel the urge to continue to eat it until that need is met, resulting in overconsumption of complex carbohydrates.

The reason most complex carbohydrates taste bland is that when you chew they break down into molecules that are too large to fit into the taste receptors in the mouth. In order to fit, a complex carbohydrate molecule has to be broken down to the size of a double sugar unit. ("Complex" carbohydrates are called complex because they are composed of more than two sugar molecule units.)

An enzyme present in saliva begins that breakdown process, but in general, complex carbohydrate molecules stay in the mouth only long enough to convert less than 5% of all their molecules into double sugar units. If you slow your chewing speed, you can increase the release of double sugar units. Further breakdown of complex carbs into double sugar units happens in the intestine, where an exocrine enzyme from the pancreas knocks the molecules apart.

What you enjoy when you eat food containing complex carbohydrates are actually the vitamins and minerals your nutrient-counting brain has come to associate with that particular carbohydrate, as well as any spices, sugar, salt, oil, or fat added to it. This means that in reality, you are enjoying only a tiny portion of the complex carbohydrates you eat. You're unlikely to be aware of this because you typically eat foods with complex carbohydrates topped with gravy, sauce, cheese, butter, syrup, jam, jelly, salt, seasonings, or other condiments. Without these, you would taste almost nothing from bread, rice, pasta, and other grain-based foods.

could be effective for a while, it may not be enough to counter cancer cells that seem to constantly devise mechanisms for evasion and escape, as they have proven to do. In addition, the intervention could cause undesirable and sometimes not immediately recognizable collateral damage along with physical, mental, and emotional toll.

As a result, the strategy I advocate is that we must focus on preventing mutated cells from multiplying so that they remain in the locality of their origin during a person's lifespan. Cancer cells can accomplish metastasis only as long as a steady supply of glucose is available for energy production. This means that they are highly vulnerable to glucose deprivation. Denying the availability of glucose can prevent almost all cancer cells from metastasis, because without glycolysis, cancer cells will have to stop their process of multiplying, moving to a new location, and starting a new colony.

Meanwhile, denying glucose to cancer cells will not impact your normal cells, especially muscle cells, as they can use fatty acids as fuel, even if you are afflicted with cancer. [53]

## Take steps to eliminate grains from your diet

If you have cancer or are concerned about developing it, it is critical to switch to a low-carbohydrate diet, largely by eliminating grains to as close to zero intake as possible. Depending on your age, especially as you approach adulthood, your body needs very little glucose, for two reasons. First, your cells multiply more slowly because new cells are mostly formed to replace dead cells within organs, rather than to build new structures. As a result, there is reduced glucose need for cell division. Then, as you age, there is usually a reduction in muscle mass, so there are fewer cells where glucose can be stored as muscle glycogen. Reduced muscle mass also means reduced energy needs.

So, how much carbohydrate should you eat? As a general rule, a healthy person can think of the answer to this question in this way: the quantity of carbohydrate consumed during a meal should be no more than what you need to replenish the glycogen stores in your liver and muscles, unless you are exercising immediately after a meal. Any excess carbohydrate that remains in the body is what your liver converts into triglycerides that get stored in your fat cells. When your fat cells are full, the excess glucose remains in your bloodstream. This means that if you tend to be sedentary, you don't need many complex carbohydrates. No one can give you a specific recommendation on quantity, but if you get in touch with your authentic weight (the weight at which your brain tells you that you are the most comfortable), you will sense how much you need to reduce your carbohydrate intake to lose weight and maintain it.

But if you have been diagnosed with cancer, your situation is completely different, as you need to cut your grain consumption to zero. To repeat, grains produce voluminous amounts of glucose that will feed your cancer cells. Begin eliminating grains from your meals, including wheat, oats, rice, barley, rye, corn, and others. It doesn't matter if it is whole grain, multi-grain, or gluten-free—*none of these help you because grain is grain is grain.*

## Feeling full without grains

Your main challenge in avoiding or reducing the amount of grain and grain-flour products will be that you may not feel that sense of having a full belly after eating. The best way to solve this is to reduce the amount you eat to one-half of what you are used to, and then reduce it down even further little by little. For example, if you are used to thick crust pizza, change to thin crust. Instead of a regular sandwich, eat an open-faced one (with one slice of bread). Later, begin eating sandwiches as lettuce wraps instead. Over time, you will learn to feel satisfied with the foods you eat, despite eating very little or no grains at all.

People of many cultures often think, "My ancestors have been eating rice or bread made with grain flour for centuries without experiencing diabetes or cancer. I grew up eating the same way and so I will feel deprived if I have to eat rice or grain-flour bread in limited quantity." Such people then ask, "Isn't there some type of grain I can consume, despite my cancer?"

To me, this is like an alcoholic asking what type of alcohol is the least damaging. The answer regarding grain and grain-flour products is it doesn't matter what your source of carbohydrate is. What matters is the total amount you consume from all food sources compared to the glycogen and fat storage capacity that you have. Any time you exceed your storage capacities you are setting yourself up for trouble. And if you have cancer, zero grain is best.

## A special note for those with Type 2 diabetes

If you are currently taking medications to control elevated blood sugar, you are going to be caught between a rock and a hard place when it comes to following the guidelines I stated above. Let me explain.

You, most likely, have been told that glucose is a very important nutrient for the body, especially for nerve cells. You may take this to mean that glucose is an essential nutrient, which it is not. In addition, you may have been warned about the dangers of low blood sugar and may have even experienced some of the symptoms of it in the form of hypoglycemia. You may have determined that you would do everything possible to avoid that situation. You may have been told not to miss meals prescribed specifically for you, to prevent low blood sugar. This, obviously, conflicts with your desire to shed some pounds to reach your authentic weight. And the longer you have been on medications to control your blood sugar, the more entrenched your eating habits have become, including the quantity of food you consume during each meal. This background may make it difficult for you to alter your eating habits. All I can tell you is that it is possible to live without grains and avoid overeating. Even those who have been on such medications for many years have successfully reduced both medications and food intake, gradually.

# What to eat

I DON'T MEAN TO SUGGEST THAT PEOPLE WHO EAT GRAINS SUCH AS rice or food items made with grain flour on a regular basis are more prone to develop cancer. You may know people in different parts of the world or your own ancestors who consumed rice, pasta, or breads daily without suffering from cancer as modern people do. If you spend the energy from the grain-products you consume for metabolic activities before your next meal, or you can store excess glucose as fat outside the bloodstream, you may be safe in consuming grain and grain-flour products. However, the fact is that the human body can survive without consuming any grains or grain-based foods.

Given that you don't need glucose from grains, and that cancer cells thrive on glucose, especially after meals loaded with carbohydrates from grains, I suggest that anyone concerned about cancer as well as all cancer survivors must have as their primary objective the avoidance of grains. This is how you can keep your blood sugar levels low at all times. It is especially important to avoid the post-prandial (after meal) elevation of sugar that helps feed cancer cells.

So what foods can you use to replace grains? Why are those foods better? That's what this section addresses.

# Eat lentils and other legumes instead of grains to help feel full

If I had to give you a single recommendation for how to eat without grains or grain products, it would be to substitute lentils into your regular diet in place of them. Lentils have been part of the human diet for almost 5,000 years. Lentils do contain carbohydrate, but they have a low "glycemic index," meaning they digest very slowly, releasing glucose little by little into the intestine and bloodstream. This reduces the availability of glucose to your cancer cells soon after a meal. In addition, just 100 grams of raw lentils can provide 50% of the Recommended Daily Intake of protein, as well as fiber and numerous fiber-associated nutrients.

Before you cook dry lentils, it can be useful to soak them in warm water overnight to reduce the amount of undesirable phytic acid that is present in many of them. Phytic acid can reduce how your body absorbs the iron and zinc in the lentils. Soaking also increases the digestibility of proteins in lentils. This is important because lentils, in general, are rich in essential amino acids.

The most common reason many people give for not eating more lentils as well as other legumes—e.g., kidney beans, black beans, garbanzo beans and other beans—is that they fear being "gassy." Beans create intestinal gas because there is a certain amount of internal fermentation of the resistant starch present in them.

But the truth is, there are several benefits to gas formation in the bowel. First, you should know that the majority of gas produced by the intestinal bacteria is absorbed into the body and expelled through the lungs. It is the remaining volume of gas that people don't like, but the fact is, this gas helps distend the intestine to start the reflex contraction needed for regular bowel movements. Without this stimulus, fecal material may not escape because there is no force to propel it forward. For example, when the consistency of fecal material is too soft, which often happens in an infection or when you have food intolerance affecting the intestine, it is the gas that helps you to eliminate the offending agent fast. In other words, gas from lentils promotes healthy elimination, a fact you probably would never have appreciated before.

# Lentils contain "resistant starch"

Lentils belong to the legume family that also includes alfalfa, clover, peas, beans, soybeans, peanuts, and tamarind.

100 grams (3.5 ounces, or slightly less than ½ a cup) of dry lentils may contain up to 60 grams of carbohydrate. However, 65 percent of this carbohydrate (about 40 grams) is in the form of "resistant starch," meaning starch that is not digestible by enzymes in the human small intestinal tract. Of the remainder, about 5% of the carbohydrate composition of lentils is readily (immediately) digestible, but the rest is digested so slowly that it is not able to cause a sudden elevation of glucose (blood sugar) that would have resulted in an insulin surge. This is why lentils are an excellent substitute for grains in meals.

In resistant starches, the carbohydrate is barely broken down by enzymes and so is not absorbed into the body through the small in-

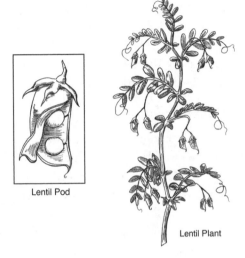

Lentil Pod

Lentil Plant

Lentils have been part of human diet for 5,000 years. Lentils digest very slowly, releasing glucose little by little into the intestine and bloodstream. Use lentils in place of a starch (rice, corn, or bread) for lunches or dinners.

testine. Instead, it passes through and reaches the large intestine (colon), where it confers benefits in the form of providing nourishment for the good bacteria there. These bacteria use the carbohydrate to produce small fatty acid compounds called *butyrate*, essential for the health and well-being of cells lining the colon. A sticky layer of mucous covers the colon lining and provides a medium for immune cells to move and do their surveillance job.

Raw lentil has about 10% dietary fiber, 25% protein and 1% fat. Lentils can provide more than 20% of the Recommended Daily Value of nutrients such as folate, thiamin, pantothenic acid, vitamin B6, phosphorus, iron, and zinc.

# The anti-cancer benefits of eating mushrooms and seaweed

Although no specific proof has been discovered regarding whether certain nutrients may prevent cancer, there is an interesting possibility that mushrooms and seaweed may have natural anti-cancer properties. Let me explain.

## Mushrooms

On the evolutionary tree, mushrooms and humans come from the same branch. Like humans, mushrooms inhale oxygen and exhale carbon dioxide. Unlike plants that get energy by photosynthesis, mushrooms use sugar and other life forms, just as we do. They adapt, live, and reproduce in diverse and even hostile environments like we do. They are known to produce a number of cell-protective antioxidants, antibacterial, and antiviral compounds and other health promoting chemicals. Some molecules from mushrooms have been found to induce cell death by activating the self-destruct mechanism in them. Some have conjugated linoleic acid that has been found to inhibit chemically induced cancer in mice.

If you decide to pick your own mushrooms, be sure to study what to pick. Each year, dozens of people experience mushroom poisoning from toxins present in certain species that are not edible and often misidentified. Some mushrooms can cause death.

## Seaweed

According to the National Ocean Service of the National Oceanic and Atmospheric Administration, many types of seaweed contain anti-inflammatory and anti-microbial agents. The ancient Romans used them to treat wounds, burns, and rashes. The ancient Egyptians may have used them as a treatment for breast cancer. Seaweed contains at least eight vitamins, eight minerals, and fiber. Japanese people have consumed seaweed for at least 1,500 years. While dietary soy has long been credited for the low rate of cancer in general in Japan, it may be that dietary seaweed is the actual indicator of robust health. Seaweed has been found to have cancer-fighting agents.[54] Antiviral compounds have been isolated from seaweed.[55]

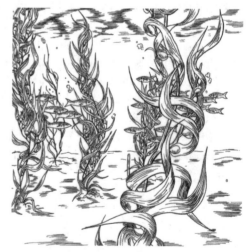

Seaweed has been found to have cancer-fighting agents. Many types of seaweed contain anti-inflammatory and anti-microbial agents, along with vitamins, minerals, and fiber. Farmed seaweed is increasingly available in the United States and can be mixed into many recipes.

# The antimicrobial power of mushrooms and seaweed

Common edible mushrooms have many natural nutrients that act as antimicrobials and stimulate the growth of immune cells. Antibiotic *ganomycin* (from reishi mushrooms) and *campestrin* (from meadow mushrooms) and the chemotherapy drugs *calvacin* (from giant puffballs) and *Illudin S* (from glow-in-the-dark jack-o'-lantern mushrooms) are examples.

In addition, *polysaccharide K*, present in some mushrooms, is found to inhibit various cancer-onset mechanisms and is being considered as an adjunct to esophageal, gastric, colorectal, breast, and lung cancer treatments.[56]

100 grams of raw brown mushrooms provide more than 20% of the Recommended Daily Value of B vitamins such as riboflavin, niacin, pantothenic acid, and dietary minerals selenium and copper. When exposed to ultraviolet light, even after harvesting, mushrooms produce vitamin D.

Certain seaweeds are found to have anticancer agents that researchers hope will prove effective in the treatment of leukemia and other cancers. Currently, seaweeds are used in many commercial products such as toothpaste, fruit jelly, cosmetics, and skin care products.

Seaweed contains carotenoids and the minerals calcium and potassium.

*Sulfated oligosaccharides* from seaweeds have been found to stimulate the growth of beneficial intestinal bacteria.[57]

Be aware, however, that rotting seaweed can produce hydrogen sulfide, which can cause vomiting and diarrhea.

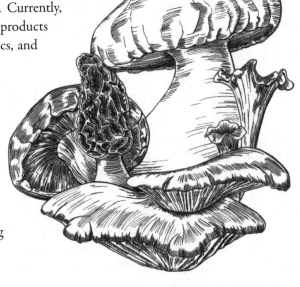

Mushrooms produce a number of cell-protective antioxidants, antibacterial, and antiviral compounds and other health promoting chemicals. Enjoy the different flavors of a wide variety of mushrooms you can find in most grocery stores.

# Consider a modified paleo diet or the ketogenic diet

There are two types of diets that might guide your thinking in how you can alter your intake of food while avoiding grains.

## Paleo diet

In recent years, the "Paleo" diet has become popular. This regimen typically focuses on eating only what our Paleolithic ancestors ate—meat, vegetables, fruits, nuts, roots. It excludes dairy products, grains, sugar, legumes, processed oils, salt, alcohol, and coffee. The thinking behind this diet is that it correlates with the foods that humans were originally intended to eat.

The Paleo diet is perhaps the closest diet to what I would recommend for people with Type 2 diabetes and/or cancer. It avoids the extensive consumption of grains that my research indicates is the cause of high blood sugar and that I believe feeds cancer cells.

Although this diet may be beneficial compared to the typical Western diet, please be aware of the potential of inadequate calcium intake when following it. Also, while very little is known about the diet of Paleolithic humans, we do know that modern humans are perfectly able to digest legumes (beans, lentils, etc.), and so I disagree that legumes should be avoided.

## Ketogenic diet

The ketogenic diet is one that emphasizes very low intake of carbohydrates and protein, and a high intake of fats. The goal of the diet is to force the body into burning fatty acids, as I have discussed, and avoid consuming glucose from carbs. The classic ketogenic diet recommends consuming a 4:1 ratio by weight of fat to combined protein and carbohydrate.

The diet is called ketogenic because when you consume a high level of fats, the liver manufactures excessive quantities of *ketone bodies* (acetoacetate and 3-hydroxybuterate) produced from the abundance of fatty acids digested from the fats. It takes a few weeks of being on this diet for the ketone bodies to appear in blood tests.

The benefit of the diet is that your muscle cells can generate energy using ketone bodies even though blood glucose levels are low. This allows you to begin starving cancer cells, thus slowing or halting their multiplication.[58] Beware, however, that if you switch to a ketogenic diet, you must be at your authentic weight with little body fat. Otherwise, if you begin releasing fatty acids from full fat cells as you lose weight, you may force normal cells to use those stored fatty acids for energy, which could make any glucose in the bloodstream available for the use of cancer cells.

# How the ketogenic diet helps your body burn fats rather than glucose

The beneficial effects of avoiding grains and grain-flour products from the diet could be taken one step further by forcing the body to burn *ketone bodies* rather than glucose to extract cellular energy. When fat cells become full, the liver is programmed to produce ketone bodies instead of triglycerides from absorbed glucose. Muscle then begins burning the ketone bodies rather than glucose. This is because ketone bodies can enter cells more easily and be reconverted into acetyl-CoA that can be captured by oxaloacetate formed in functioning mitochondria, as long as oxygen is available.

The metabolism of ketone bodies is a normal, physiological function of the body, thanks to our inheritance of an adaptive mechanism for survival during periods of prolonged starvation such as famines experienced by our ancestors. The primary objective of this adaptive mechanism is to spare muscle proteins from degradation. Without this mechanism, control centers in the brain needing glucose as the fuel will command the liver to produce glucose using amino acids from any source, including muscle proteins. You may survive a famine but could be too weak to function afterwards. However, the ability of cells, including nerve cells, to use ketone bodies to produce fuel results in the utilization of fat for fuel, sparing muscle protein from destruction.[59]

You go on a ketogenic diet to starve cancer cells of glucose. However, if you cheat and consume carbohydrates, be aware that cancer cells are unaffected by the simple presence of ketone bodies. In other words, it is not the presence of ketones itself that inhibits the proliferation of cancer cells; it is the absence of glucose, as seen in animal studies. *[60]

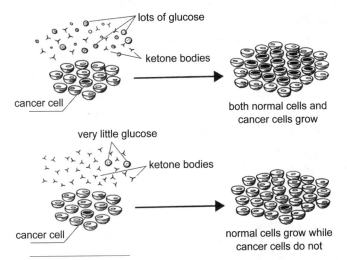

lots of glucose

ketone bodies

cancer cell

both normal cells and cancer cells grow

very little glucose

ketone bodies

cancer cell

normal cells grow while cancer cells do not

(Top) Going on a ketogenic diet does not help if you continue to have high blood sugar. Both normal and cancer cells can use the glucose for growth. (Bottom) However, in the presence of very little glucose, normal cells can grow using the ketone bodies for energy but cancer cells will not since they are deprived of glucose.

---

* Proof of this can be found in an experiment in which cells from a human brain tumor (glioma) were implanted into mice brain. After the viability of tumor cells was established, the control group was given a standard diet containing 55% carbohydrate by weight while the study group was given a ketogenic diet containing 0.2% carbohydrate. Cancer cells were not able to multiply when deprived of glucose but treated with ketone bodies as a substitute for glucose, whereas normal nerve cells were able to survive with energy from ketone bodies even when starved of glucose.[61]

# Can you eat specific nutrients to prevent cancer?

Nutrients needed by cancer cells are the same as those needed by normal cells. So, how do you choose nutrition therapy to help normal cells without helping cancer cells? The answer is, it's complicated and you have to be careful.

For example, you should be aware that a detected deficiency of a nutrient might not be the actual *cause* of the cancer, but rather an indication that cancer cells are actually using that nutrient for their sustenance.

For instance, you might detect a low level of folic acid in the blood, because cancer cells in the bone marrow are using it to proliferate. However, if you think that low folic acid caused the formation of cancer cells in the bone marrow and supplement your diet with folic acid in an attempt to correct the deficiency, you could actually stimulate faster cancer growth. On the other hand, high folate intake has been found to be associated with a lower incidence of breast cancer in postmenopausal women.[62] So as you can see, it is not clear-cut.

Nevertheless, it is possible that a needed nutrient can be useful in altered form to stop the growth of cancer. We do know that many naturally occurring chemicals found in plants appear to block the activity of cancer promoters. We can only hope that in the future, we will learn more about the nutrient profile of particular cancers so that they could be mapped out. This might allow us to develop specific diets that emphasize those nutrients as the way to halt the cancer.

Meanwhile, in my view, you should focus on eating a wide variety of foods to ensure that you obtain as many nutrients as possible. If you think about it, every human, regardless of the region of Earth where they live, needs the same nutrients to survive. And the fact that people live nearly everywhere on Earth means that those nutrients are generally available from whatever foods are locally grown and raised where they live.

With approximately 220 different types of cells in the body, and new cells being formed from stem cells on a continuous basis to complement existing cells or to replace dead cells, the body needs a wide assortment of nutrients on a continuous basis. These nutrients are necessary to maintain the integrity of cell structure, and to perform the specialized functions of each organ or tissue of which the cell is a part. For example, the formation of red blood cells needs iron, that of bones needs calcium, and retinal cells of the eye need vitamin A. Therefore, it is imperative to maintain those nutrients in the fluid outside those cells in a desired range to sustain life through the development, growth, and maintenance of normal body cells. The same is, of course, true for all cells in other organs of the body.

The objective of nourishment is thus to make it possible for the body to take care of itself, and probably protect itself from cancer as well. Eating vegetables as fresh as possible is the best way to get cancer-protective nutrients from the food you eat. Vegetables grown without herbicides and pesticides will naturally contain molecules they self-manufacture to protect themselves from invaders. Eating and absorbing these molecules helps humans boost their own immune system that evolved for thousands of years based on instructions received from plant-based molecules.

# Benefits of nutritional therapy

There are many diets claiming to help you avoid cancer using various vitamins, minerals, or protective plant compounds containing phytochemicals that help defend the body against cancer. In addition, individual nutrients are widely marketed as agents that will help prevent cancer, manage its symptoms, or improve the immune system. However, you have to keep in mind that there are not many controlled studies to back up such health claims.

In order to be proven as a protective cancer agent, the absence of a nutrient has to be shown to cause cancer. This is extremely difficult to research and prove. Even if this were possible to do in animals, it does not automatically mean that cancer of the same cell in humans is caused by the same mechanism, since many gene interactions play an important role in cancer formation.

Ultimately, the beneficial role that your nutrition plays in the presence of cancer cells can be viewed in two ways: 1) to boost your immune system, and 2) to support the normal cells in the body. These roles can be complicated when someone is using chemotherapy, radiation, surgery, and other interventions, as these treatments could produce a number of side effects, including decreased appetite. Therefore, if you are undergoing one of these treatments, in addition to frequent meals, nutritional supplementation should also be considered.

In addition, special care should be taken to consume foods that contain the necessary ingredients for the manufacture of new cells, especially if you have had chemotherapy that resulted in destruction of cell lines that need to be reconstituted. This includes foods that contain essential fatty acids, such as walnuts, pumpkin seeds, sunflower seeds, fish, and shellfish. You also will need all necessary amino acids in the right ratio, and these can be obtained by consuming egg whites or whey protein.

Even if you end up modifying some of their nutrients by cooking, eating a varied plant-based diet is better than consuming a tablet, liquid, or a specific food advertised as an "immune booster." In my view, eating fresh, seasonal foods that can enhance the immune system is far healthier for anyone with cancer than any type of processed or pre-packaged food that is supposed to boost your immune system. Another reason for this is that it is impossible to identify and completely avoid any cancer-promoting contaminants in pre-packaged foods.

Various studies have shown that a prudent dietary pattern characterized by high intakes of fruits, vegetables, legumes, low-fat dairy products, poultry, and fish was associated with a decreasing risk of overall death. However, nutritional therapy has not been proven to halt mortality from cancer.

# The health benefits of cooking with fresh herbs and spices

We've been discussing extensively that it is important for you to eat a variety of foods to obtain all the nutrients that your body needs to remain healthy. An additional recommendation that I suggest in this regard is to cook with fresh or dried herbs and spices as often as you get a chance to do so. Recent studies have associated consuming spiced foods for 1 or 2 days a week with lower risk of death, as well as a lower risk of diseases such as cancer, compared to not eating them.

Why do spices help? Some investigators have suggested that fresh spices make available important nutrients such as vitamins A, K, and B6. In addition, spices such as turmeric, ginger, capsaicin, and anethole (anise camphor) have been credited with anticancer properties.[63] Many other herbs and spices are being looked at as adjuvants (helpers) capable of ameliorating symptoms associated with cancer.

Note that some spices must be paired with others to be effective for the body. For instance, curcumin from turmeric may not be absorbed in significant amounts unless it is paired with ginger or pepper.

In addition, spices can be helpful to regulate your food intake if the same types and similar amounts of spices are used during the preparation of a specific dish. By reinforcing the enjoyment of eating a particular food, over time spices may act as signal-amplifying agents for your brain to create the sense of satisfaction that leads you to stop eating when the intensity of the taste noticeably subsides. This helps you avoid overeating.

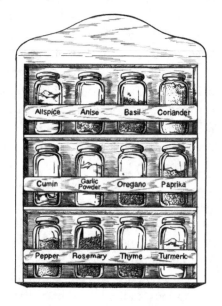

I would recommend trying to get your fill of micronutrients from fresh herbs and spices rather than in pill or liquid form as supplements. These supplements may not help because they sometimes do not contain sufficient quantities of the product, or they contain ingredients not listed on the label, or they contain much more of a nutrient than needed. And an extract cannot simply be a stand-in because a purified extract may have different effects than the whole herb.

Finally, note that not all spices are "spicy." Many spices simply add a different flavor, without making it "hot" in the mouth. They do not make your tongue tingle or your mouth feel on fire. Their role is simply to add to the delicious flavor of the food in a pleasant way, or to add appealing color.

# Spices contain many micro-nutrients your body needs

The foods humans eat contain both macronutrients and micronutrients. Our hunter-gatherer ancestors may have had to travel to many different areas to obtain food, especially micronutrients. They may also have been compelled to eat more foods containing macronutrients such as carbohydrates, protein, and fats just to get enough of the needed micronutrients.

The need for micronutrients can lead to a circular problem of eating too much food. For example, when you eat an energy-containing food such as grits to obtain the micronutrient niacin, your body has to handle the other nutrients in grits. This means the body will be seeking more micronutrients to metabolize the extra carbohydrate the body absorbs from the grits. Your brain, in turn, may prod you to eat even more.

One way to get around this vicious cycle is by finding an alternate source for micronutrients. One of the best sources of these is natural spices and herbs that come from different parts of plants. This may be why the use of spices and herbs in cooking started as far back as at least 2000 BCE, as early humans may have realized that spices not only made food taste better, but that they could eat less food and still obtain their energy needs.

Spices have also long been used to preserve food for long periods of time. While our ancestors did not understand the reason, the antimicrobial properties make spices a useful food ingredient, especially in warmer climates, where infectious diseases can be spread through meat, which is particularly susceptible to spoiling. However, this doesn't explain the extensive use of spices in a country like India, where much of the population is vegetarian, or their use in Mediterranean cultures that use a lot of fresh seafood.

My explanation for mankind's use of spices in cooking comes back to the brain's regulatory mechanism that we have discussed. I suggest that spices are used to make meals more enjoyable because, in the brain, this enjoyment signifies the arrival of a needed micronutrient in the mouth. The evidence for this lies in the fact that spices and herbs contain abundant vitamins, minerals, and antioxidants in significant portions that make them ideal sources of micronutrients. In fact, herbs and spices can be the source of at least 25% of the 118+ nutrients that scientists have so far identified as necessary for the body.

The World Cancer Research Foundation 2007 report estimated that 35% of the cancer incidence worldwide could be attributable to lifestyle factors, including food. A diet protective against cancer would include spices. For example, the United States was found to have much higher rates of colorectal cancer compared to that cancer's incidence in India. The high consumption of spices is thought to be one of the contributing factors in the lower number of colon cancer cases reported in India.[64]

Humans have been using spices for well over 5,000 years. The potential of their beneficial effect on prevention and treatment of cancer has been investigated over the last several decades. Using rodents in experimental settings has shown encouraging results. Yet, in spite of over 100 clinical trials with spices and their components in human subjects, we still need confirmatory evidence to clearly understand their beneficial effect in surviving cancer.

## Can I eat refined sugar?

Refined sugar is not the same as blood sugar. Glucose is the form of sugar in blood sugar—the fuel for cells. Cancer cells thrive on glucose. The sugar you consume in various foods is *sucrose* (refined sugar), or *lactose* (milk sugar), or *fructose* (fruit sugar). High-fructose corn syrup, which is often added to juices, sodas and fruity yogurts, is 55% fructose and 45% glucose.

Sucrose is derived from various sources such as sugarcane, which has been grown and refined in India since 500 BCE. It can also come from sugar beets. Juices from these plants produce refined sugar. The industrial revolution in America and Europe made it easy for many foods containing refined sugar, including confectionary and desserts, to be mass produced, processed, preserved, canned, packaged, advertised, sold, and consumed.

So what is the role of sucrose in health and well-being, and its effect on cancer? The first answer is that it is not the type of sugar that is important but the total quantity of carbohydrate in the intestine from foods you eat that results in the elevation of blood sugar when the carbohydrate is absorbed into the body. So keeping your intake of sucrose down is important, though not as critical as avoiding grains.

That said, keep in mind that refined sugar has often been blamed for the prevalence of obesity, Type 2 diabetes, and other health problems. However, there are no studies showing any health benefits from avoiding refined sugar, even for those diagnosed with Type 2 diabetes.

Nevertheless, I would not recommend consuming much refined sugar for the following reason. Most refined sugar is consumed in products containing grains and grain-flour—pies, cakes, muffins, candies, and other sweet desserts, plus it is often found in canned products.

My position is that the natural sugar present in whole fruits or vegetables is far less of a health risk compared to grain and grain-flour products consumed on a daily basis, often multiple times.

# The plague of high sugar-content drinks

There is a literal pandemic of beverages and foods now produced with added sugar or high-fructose corn syrup. These are well-known taste-enhancing additives that increase the palatability, presentation, aroma, and texture of food to make consumers want to eat more than they need in a serving.

The proof of this is in the astonishing statistic that Americans consume an average of 22 teaspoons of added sugar per day, most of it in the form of soda and sweetened drinks. You may not realize the enormous amount of sugar in many of these drinks. While an eight-ounce glass of milk contains about three teaspoons of natural sugar, there are eight teaspoons of sugar in a can of regular soda.

These beverages are often consumed in response to thirst when the brain expects receptors in the mouth to experience water molecules. If the sugar concentration in such beverages were similar to that of a natural beverage, such as milk, the body would be able to regulate the sugar consumed. But if the beverage you consume is sweetened with sugar or an energy-containing sweetener at a concentration above what is natural, the brain has no mechanism to regulate how much you need to drink to satisfy your thirst based on the experience of sweet taste. You are then forced to terminate drinking based either on a feeling of fullness in your stomach or the emptiness of the container.

This is why many people tend to drink large amounts of soft drinks or sweetened juices when they are thirsty, adding to their increased consumption of sugar. I recommend weaning yourself off sodas and beverages with added sugar or high-fructose corn syrup to reduce your intake of carbohydrates. Even more important is to preserve your brain's natural mechanism to regulate your nutrient intake based on sensing sweetness just as nature produces in fresh fruits and vegetables.

# The importance of the bacteria in your gut

The human body harbors about 100 trillion bacteria, outnumbering human cells 10 to 1. Every square centimeter of your skin may have about a hundred thousand bacteria eating the flakes of skin you shed. They also drink the water coming out of the pores in the skin. In addition to the bacteria you nourish with skin flakes while you are awake, you feed up to two million microscopic mites that resides in your mattress and pillows with skin flakes you shed as you sleep.

However, the most important bacteria may be the ones residing in the gut, which contains several hundred types. Is there one that nature intended to be the most beneficial?

A clue can be obtained from the intestinal bacteria of breast-fed infants. As you can imagine, many bacteria will enter the mouth of a human baby. Most will perish by the actions of stomach acid and digestive enzymes in the small intestine. But those that survive start colonizing the gut quickly, as a single bacterium can produce billions of copies in a single day. The ones that reach the lower intestine must be able to survive in an environment almost completely deprived of oxygen and have the ability to produce energy needed for their survival and reproduction using what is left of the breast milk after the digestive enzymes in the small intestine have acted on it. The winner is *Bifidobacterium*, a bacterial variety that not only survives in a low-oxygen environment but thrives in it.

One of the reasons to eat a wide variety of foods is thus to feed the good bacteria in the gut. Not only do these bacteria help with digestion of food, they are also critical to your immune system's white blood cells, which are in charge of protecting your body from invaders such as germs and cancer cells. Immune cells passing through the colon are thus trained to accept normal colon bacteria as a part of you.

In a symbiotic relationship, intestinal bacteria and humans benefit from each other. While bacteria get a secure, warm, nutrient-rich, and oxygen-free place in the gut to survive, they help the body in different ways. A protected and healthy colony of the resident bacteria produce *butyrate*, a fatty acid compound that provides nourishment for the cells lining the colon. Without butyrate for their energy production, these cells can't survive. An unhealthy lining can succumb to ingested cancer-causing chemicals. In addition, butyrate inhibits the activity of immune cells that can cause chronic inflammation in the colon. Butyrate also plays a role in suppressing the growth of blood vessels induced by signals from cancer cells.

# Bacteria: Sentinels in the intestine

Bifidobacteria consume the sugar called *oligosaccharide*, among the most common solid components of breast milk, and not digestible by enzymes in the small intestine. Breast milk contains over 150 varieties of human milk oligosaccharides (and these are not present in infant formula). In older infants that begin to eat solid foods, Bifidobacteria digest plant-based oligosaccharides that are much smaller, containing 3 to 9 simple glucose molecules (compared to up to 200,000 molecules of glucose found in each molecule of complex carbohydrate in grains and grain-based foods).

In adults, the "resistant" carbohydrate contained in lentils is a good source of food for Bifidobacteria. The other source is yacon, a tuber commonly cultivated in the Peruvian Andes. It has a higher percentage of oligosaccharides that become available to the Bifidobacteria in the colon, compared to most other items in adult food.

In healthy humans, Bifidobacterium bacteria produce *conjugated linoleic acid* (CLA). There is some evidence that CLA may have anti-cancer properties, but there is no clear evidence in humans. In addition, one or more oligosaccharides joined to a protein on the outer side of the cell membrane create decoy receptors for disease-causing bacteria, and aid immune cells to spot the unwanted bacteria. Immune cells are trained to scan the receptors to detect alterations of the attachment between oligosaccharide and a given protein. This helps them determine the nature of an invader or the potential for cancer development.

## CURIOUS TIDBITS

The human blood groups (O, A, B) are determined in part by the nature of the oligosaccharide attached to proteins on the blood cell membrane.

# Another reason to keep your colon healthy

A healthy colon contains good bacteria that produce vitamins B and K that can be absorbed into the body. Good bacteria also convert dietary compounds to usable molecules, neutralize the pro-cancer activities of harmful bacteria, and metabolize natural compounds that could cause unwanted biological activities. Such compounds may have entered the body from animals or fish consumed from rivers and streams that contain bacteria or sewage that was discarded or flushed into the water.

But in addition to providing a home for good bacteria, a healthy colon provides another protective mechanism for fighting cancer—its lining. A healthy lining prevents the entry of toxic products from infective agents that may colonize the gut, or from cancer-causing chemicals introduced in the foods you consume. Mucous released by the colon lining plays important functions as a lubricant for the smooth passage of waste as well as a facilitator for the transport of enzyme molecules and cells. Meanwhile, while traversing the colon during their training and surveillance activities, immune cells adhere to the mucous and are not swept out of the body during elimination, thus preserving their presence to scout for invaders.

Healthy colon mucous also protects the intestinal lining from the action of digestive enzymes entering from the small intestine, all the while allowing the butyrate and other small fatty acid compounds produced by bacteria to diffuse into the colon lining. While a healthy lining facilitates entry of nutrients into the body, healthy mucous provides protection for the colon lining.

Finally, an intact and healthy intestinal barrier also prevents invading pathogens and ingested toxins from promoting inflammatory responses in the gut. Patients with an unhealthy lining are more likely to have inflammatory bowel disease and a higher risk of colorectal cancer compared to healthy populations.[65]

The most striking example of the protective power of the intestinal lining is the condition called "necrotizing enterocolitis" experienced by premature babies, who because of prematurity have not developed a fully functional lining in the colon. By providing the baby with healthy bacteria—probiotics and food those bacteria eat (prebiotic)—many babies have been able to manufacture the healthy lining and survive. One of the most undervalued benefits of breast-feeding is thus the protection of the intestinal lining and establishment of a healthy colony of gut bacteria.

In short, a healthy gut lined with healthy cells producing healthy mucous and colonized by healthy bacteria is essential for a healthy life.

# The gut as training ground for white blood cells

Although humans rely on oxygen for producing the energy needed for metabolic activities, 99% of the bacteria in the gut do not require oxygen for survival. In fact, they may die in the presence of oxygen. This provides an ideal training ground for white cells for target practice because they actually release oxygen to kill invading bacteria.

Among the ten million varieties of white cells, each specialized to identify a particular target, are also lymphocytes, which are tasked with identifying normal cells versus intruders or damaged cells. When lymphocytes encounter invasive bacteria detrimental to the existence of normal gut bacteria, they will seek to destroy them. Recognizing the telltale protein of the invader, lymphocytes inform the nearest immune surveillance facility—the lymph node—to send reinforcements to neutralize the offending agent.

Most white cells last only a short time, from a few hours to a few days. However, there is a class of "memory" lymphocytes—cells that have previously encountered invaders such as bacteria, viruses, and cancer cells. Based on their prior exposure, they can mount a faster and stronger immune response when they encounter the same situation again.

When memory cells have to be replaced due to old age, the newly minted lymphocytes need to be trained. Where can newly-produced immune cells be trained to recognize normal cells versus invaders? The answer is, at the school of bacteria in the gut.

The problem is, when newly minted memory lymphocyte cells are sent to the gut for training to recognize normal cells that are part of every organ in the body, sometimes the process can misfire. This is one of the causes of an autoimmune response, when immune cells attack normal cells in the body.

# Do you need to supplement with dietary fiber?

Dietary fiber refers to edible parts of plants and can be eaten directly. It has two main components.

- *Insoluble fiber* is not digestible by enzymes in the small intestine but provides bulk by absorbing water from the intestinal wall. Insoluble fiber provides nourishment for bacteria in the large intestine.

- *Soluble fiber* is readily fermented in the colon to physiologically active products that are beneficial to the body. In addition, gases generated during fermentation are absorbed into the body to be released through the lungs, the rectum, or compressed to reach the level of pressure necessary to initiate elimination of waste from the body. This could be the reason why not eating enough vegetable fibers, for the needed bulk, or not providing nutrition to the right type of bacteria in the gut to produce enough gas, leads to chronic constipation in some people.

Many products are on the market claiming to contain beneficial fiber, including reducing the risk of colon cancer. There is evidence suggesting that consumption of fiber may offer the benefit of protecting against risk of progressing from prediabetes to Type 2 diabetes. Fiber might do this by delaying post-prandial (after meals) glucose absorption.

However, dietary supplementation with fiber has not been clinically proven to be beneficial in controlled studies. For example, the authors of a study using flaxseed for glycemic control observed lower A1C blood tests when people had a low-dose intervention of flaxseed. However, paradoxically, there was no change when people were given a high dose of flaxseed. The authors also could not explain the absence of improvement in fasting *fructosamine* values (another marker of glycemic control based on glycated albumin) at low and high dose supplementation.[66]

One caution to watch out for: Many of the dietary fibers supposedly in some products are not actually fibrous.

Natural nuts, seeds, and legumes such as beans and peas are the most convenient and easily available sources of dietary fiber—eating them is the solution I recommend.

# Does a high fiber diet help fight cancer or any disease?

The digestion of food resulting in the release and absorption of nutrients into the body happens in the small intestine. Enzymes in charge of digestion in the small intestine need sufficient time, as is the case with all enzymatic actions. The presence of indigestible vegetable fiber helps slow the movement of food through the small intestine for this to happen. In addition, it takes time for vegetable fibers to bind to bile acids, which helps lower the reabsorption of cholesterol into the body.

Although the body's usual objective is to eliminate waste as soon as possible, since each meal can result in the production of waste, you don't want to be in a position to have to go to the bathroom after each meal. The large intestine serves as a safe holding area until the body is ready to eliminate, unless, of course, there is urgency such as in an infection, food intolerance, or allergy. This waiting period is the time for intestinal bacteria to produce the needed amount of gas to stretch the intestinal wall to promote laxation. In addition, bacterial action produces fatty acids that balance intestinal acidity, impact gene expression, and improve immune function, all of which are important processes in reducing the risk of colon cancer.

## Other benefits of high fiber diet on the body

A nine-year study of 388,000 adults ages 50 to 71 found that the highest consumers of vegetable fiber were at lower risk of from heart disease, infectious and respiratory illnesses, and cancer-related death.[67] Current recommendations from the United States National Academy of Sciences suggest that adults should consume 20-35 grams of dietary fiber per day. Unfortunately, the average American's daily intake of dietary fiber is only 12-18 grams. So, be sure to eat more fiber.

# Reduce your alcohol consumption (sorry, but it's true)

The American Society of Clinical Oncology recommends avoiding alcoholic drinks to reduce the risk of cancer because the risk of developing several types of cancer increases with the amount of alcohol consumed.[68]

However, what is not clear is the degree of contribution from alcohol compared to other cancer-causing agents from the environment and food you consume. For example, even those who don't drink alcohol can develop cancer. This means that the exact way that alcohol causes or increases the risk of cancer has not been completely understood. One possibility is repeated cell injury caused by prolonged, heavy drinking. This results in an accelerated cell regeneration, which leads to the potential for mutations. The increased risk of cancer in patients with cirrhosis of the liver supports this possibility. In addition, a higher risk of cancers of the mouth, esophagus, throat, colon, and rectum is seen in alcohol users than in non-alcohol users.

Another point to keep in mind: Unlike the lining of the intestine, which is designed for absorption, the lining of the stomach resists penetration of nutrients and other agents, except for two substances: alcohol and aspirin. Both of these can penetrate the barrier and cause damage. Repeated destruction of the lining of the stomach wall leads to the condition called chronic gastritis. While this is not cancer, it can become a severe condition that impacts one's ability to digest.

In addition, some alcohol users also suffer a condition called chronic pancreatitis. Combined, chronic gastritis and chronic pancreatitis interfere with the normal production, release, and action of a number of digestive enzymes produced and released by the stomach and pancreas. This can result in up to a third of carbohydrate consumed reaching the colon without being absorbed, causing fermentation and alcohol production by the intestinal bacteria.

In other words, alcohol molecules can be in the body even if you don't consume food or beverages containing alcohol, because organisms in your intestine produce them and they are absorbed into the blood. Alcohol molecules can attach to other molecules, causing changes in configuration and functionality.

Also, chemicals getting attached to alcohol may have entered the body through the mouth, skin, or mucous membrane. This makes it impossible to separate the role of drinking alcohol from that of ingested alcohol-associated chemicals in cancer formation, unless a specific mechanism can be demonstrated.

However, for men over 50 and women over 60, the cardiovascular benefits of drinking red wine in moderation may outweigh the risks of cancer.

# The link between cancer and grilled food + alcohol

If you have heard that grilled foods can cause cancer, here is the link that explains how and why.

The chemical benzopyrene is released in the environment from wood burning, in grilled foods such as grilled meats and, of course, in tobacco smoke. Anyone eating grilled foods will ingest some level of the chemical. The problem is, benzopyrene is detoxified in the liver by enzymes that also detoxify alcohol and some medications such as barbiturates. The presence of significant amounts of alcohol may result in the incomplete detoxification of benzopyrene, with some of its metabolites binding to DNA. This can cause mutations and eventually cancer.

Does this mean you should not drink alcohol if you are grilling food? The verdict is not certain because of the unpredictability of the degree of mutations an individual can experience from exposure to multiple agents.

# What to drink to support your health during cancer

Eating consciously, slowly, and mindfully is the best way to get all nutrients needed at the right amounts for optimal functioning of the body. This is accomplished easier if you drink plain water during meals. Plain water cleans your taste buds after you swallow each bite of well-chewed food by removing nutrients already on the taste receptors. If you do not like to drink plain cold water, warm it up or even flavor it with tea, mint, ginger, lemon grass, or another natural herbal flavor.

The goal is to allow the nutrients in the food to register with your taste buds and smell receptors that connect with your brain's regulatory system to monitor your food intake. Clean taste buds also allow nutrients released during the process of chewing to be recognized, which stimulates your memory of eating that food and increases your enjoyment of it. Meanwhile, the warm air going up the back of your throat, after sipping warm water, will clean the smell receptors, allowing you to enjoy the fat-associated nutrients released during chewing.

If you are experiencing dryness of the mouth or skin due to chemotherapy, you may need to consume more plain water than you normally would.

Stay away from water sweetened with any non-energy-containing sweetener (i.e., artificial sweeteners not containing natural sugar) because the manufactured intensity of sweetness can make it difficult for your brain's control centers to function properly to regulate your food intake. The brain's natural regulatory mechanism is based on the intensity of sweetness found in nature. When the brain recognizes a naturally sweet taste, it knows that the sensation means the intestine will absorb some energy-containing nutrients very soon.

But when you drink artificially sweetened drinks, which deliver no energy-containing nutrients to the intestines within the expected time, your brain may be forced to change the meaning of the sensation of sweet taste. If you drink artificially sweetened drinks over long periods of time, your brain may lose its ability to assess the meaning of sweetness even from naturally sweet items such as fruits.

## The benefits of natural plant nutrients

Scientists have identified natural plant nutrients called phytochemicals having the property to defend the body from toxins before they cause cell damage that may lead to cancer, or capable of stopping cancer cell multiplication. You can maximize the intake of these protective phytochemicals by choosing a variety of vegetables: dark leafy greens, tomatoes, carrots, and other colorful produce. However, don't be tempted to load up on phytochemicals by drinking vegetable juice preparations, even those made with 100% natural ingredients. The problem is that quantity control is difficult to measure, as you have a tendency to overconsume juices.

# Eating less as you age

You will be amazed, as you pass age 40, how little food you need during any given meal to sustain yourself until the next meal, unless your job requires strenuous physical activity. Most adults typically need less food because they usually become less active. As you age, you also begin losing muscle mass, meaning you literally can't burn fuel to produce energy as you could in your younger days.

But please note: while you need fewer calories, you still require the same quality and diversity of nutrients as you did when you were younger. Since no one else but you can know your nutrient needs, you have to rely on your own internal monitoring and metering mechanisms to ensure you consume adequate amounts of nutrients during meals.

This means your brain's ability to assess the nutrition in your food is directly proportional to the amount of time nutrients remain in contact with your taste and smell receptors. The more time you keep nutrients in contact with them, by chewing slowly, the more signals your brain receives—and the more enjoyment of food you have. In short, reducing the quantity of food you consume need not translate into the reduced pleasure of eating.

In addition, note that people who eat spiced foods do not have to consume a lot of energy nutrients to get many of the essential nutrients they need. If you eat a meal cooked with spices, you will not only enjoy the taste, but may feel satisfied with less quantity of food because the spices provide you with needed micronutrients.

Your mission during a meal should be to eat what you enjoy and, more importantly, to enjoy what you eat. Keep in mind that enjoyment is based on awareness of what is in your mouth and not proportional to the quantity consumed.

# How nature helps us to eat less

The mouth has between 2,000 and 5,000 taste buds located on the tongue, roof, sides, and back of the mouth, and in the throat. The sensation of taste includes sweetness, sourness, saltiness, bitterness, and umami (savoriness, such as found in mushrooms, cheeses, and anchovies). The flavor of a food is also affected by smell, texture, temperature, coolness, and pungency of the item being consumed. The importance that evolution has attributed to the function of our taste and smell receptors is evidenced by the fact that they are frequently replaced as they wear out.

The importance of taste buds in the regulation of nutrient intake is dramatically evident in the condition called Addison's disease. People who are affected cannot maintain proper sodium levels in the blood because of impaired kidney function in retaining sodium. However, as long as their salt-sensing taste receptors are in working order, they can maintain blood salt levels in the normal range if they have access to foods that are classified as too salty by people who are not affected by this condition. Their taste buds help them regulate their salt intake.

One of the ways nature helps us downsize our food intake, as we get older, is by reducing the total number of taste buds starting around 50 years of age. This could be one of the reasons those who live in nursing homes eat less and do not gain weight or become diabetics, despite doing less and less physical activity. However, many people override what nature is trying to do by (1) eating on a schedule rather than based on demand as exhibited by their own sensations of hunger; (2) eating a certain volume of food rather than terminating their meals based on feeling a sense of satisfaction; and (3) consuming food that requires very little or no chewing.

# Weight, body fat, and exercise

WHAT ARE THE ROLES OF WEIGHT GAIN, ACCUMULATION OF BODY fat, and exercise in surviving cancer? The question is important because as we age people tend to gain weight and become more sedentary. Since the incidence of cancer increases as we get older, something we can't escape, let us better understand the importance of weight maintenance and losing fat, and that of exercise, to formulate an action plan.

In adults, being overweight is defined as the accumulation of fat that has taken place after childhood. In general, enough fat is stored in a normal-weight adult to provide fuel to maintain a basal rate of metabolism for three months. The amount of body fat has been determined to be a better predictor of health risk than total body weight. In fact, excess body fat is now recognized as a contributing factor to the toll of cancer on Americans, ahead of tobacco.

In this section, we will look at how to reconnect with your authentic weight, lose pounds if necessary, and what role exercise may play in surviving cancer.

# Lose body fat and reconnect with your authentic weight

If you have been diagnosed with cancer, it is important to reconnect with what I call your "authentic weight." I believe most people intuitively know what their authentic weight should be. It is generally the weight you were at when you were in your mid-20s. (Scientifically speaking, your authentic weight is when your blood test values of fasting glucose, triglyceride, and cholesterol are within the normal range. This can be assessed by a blood test.) Of course, you can also look in the mirror and see whether you are carrying layers of fat in your abdomen, hips, or buttocks.

More than half of a typical person's body fat accumulates around the midsection. This is not surprising considering the fact that this is the pattern most babies follow in their first year of life. If you look at toddlers, you will see they often have a potbelly, created from the accumulation of fat converted from food consumed but not used for metabolic activity. It is thus not surprising that adults follow this same pattern, storing most of their fat in their belly. However, unlike a toddler who eventually uses this fat for vertical growth, about half of adults in the United States keep it on forever.

Paying attention to your authentic weight is your brain's way of signaling that you are healthy, or that you are exceeding the weight that is right for you. If you are in tune with your authentic weight, you immediately sense it when you gain a few extra pounds, as you start to feel uncomfortable. Your stomach may feel bloated, you may feel some muscle pains, or you may feel slower and more tired. Exceeding your authentic weight may prompt you to become aware that you need to lose some pounds.

The reason you want to be at your authentic weight is that this is the point at which you probably have the least amount of body fat. Excess body fat is associated with the risk of cancer at several organ sites, including colon and breast.[69] Growth promoters released by fat cells filled to capacity are thought to increase the risk of breast cancer in women with low estrogen concentrations (such as post-menopausal women not receiving replacement therapy). Excess body fat accounts for as many as 84,000 cancer diagnoses each year, according to the National Cancer Institute, resulting in 14% of all deaths from cancer in men and 20% of those in women. Epidemiological studies indicate that the progression of cancer increases even faster when obesity is compounded by Type 2 diabetes.[70]

This advice is especially important for women because body fat is the main site of estrogen synthesis when the ovaries cease their production, and it is also directly associated with high circulating insulin levels.[71] Both estrogen and insulin promote cancer cell multiplication. In addition, full fat cells release signaling molecules that tell the body to create more fat cells, so gaining weight effectively becomes a self-promoting process, until your body has no more fat stem cells.

# The ineffectiveness of commercial weight loss programs

Most weight loss programs base their recommendations on the assumption that how much you should eat is governed by your body's energy needs, despite your pangs of hunger. In these programs, losing weight can thus be accomplished by reducing one's consumption of energy-containing nutrients. Your body will then draw its energy from your stores of fat cells, and you lose weight.

Theoretically, this seems to make sense, but it is not entirely correct. It is true that reducing consumption—i.e., eating fewer calories—can cause your body to burn fat. However, in practice, unless you have been fasting for many days, most overweight people will have enough energy stores of fat to remain overweight for a long time. If you consider that one pound of fat represents 3,500 calories, you have to burn a huge amount of calories to lose any significant weight. And while losing this fat may eventually occur, you will probably continue to be hungry and, unless you are committed to fasting, you will experience the natural urge to eat.

What you need to understand is that the body's hunger signals reflect the fact that your brain detects a need for nutrients that your cells require for many types of metabolic activities. In other words, when your body needs nutrients, it will announce it to you via the hunger signal. This is why diet programs don't work—people still need to eat to supply their cells with needed nutrients in a timely fashion.

The best way to lose weight and maintain reduced weight is to listen to your own body by following these guidelines: Eat only in response to hunger, eat a variety of minimally processed foods that require chewing, stop eating when you are satisfied rather than wait until you feel full, and take time to enjoy each bite of food.

### CURIOUS TIDBITS

Your total body weight is the sum of the many elements in your body, including your muscles, bones, organs, fat, and also fluids. Many people think they can assess whether they are overweight using "standardized" weight charts or the Body Mass Index, but these are actually inaccurate. Weight tables have groupings that are as wide as 20 pounds, so you cannot be sure whether you should be at the lower end or higher end of the range based on your height and age. You might be carrying an additional 15 pounds while believing you are "within your range." BMI charts compensate for height but can't distinguish between muscle, bone, fat, and water weight. The best approximation of your authentic weight is your body weight when your blood glucose and triglyceride levels are at normal levels.

# Is it useful to count calories to lose weight?

I do not believe that it is useful to count calories for the purpose of losing weight. When you eat in response to hunger, it is because your brain has received messages from cells indicating that various nutrients are missing and needed. If you select your foods based on calorie counting, you may be depriving your body of nutrients that your cells need.

The only exception to this is when you have cancer and you are seeking to lose weight. In this case, it may be useful to use calories as a measure of your energy intake. In addition to avoiding grains and grain-based foods, you should also reduce total energy intake. A two-year randomized controlled trial in 218 young and middle-aged healthy normal-weight and moderately overweight men and women who achieved 12% calorie restriction below their usual intake, sustained for the entire length of the study, showed metabolic benefits, as follows:

- an average loss of 10 percent of the body weight
- a lowering of average blood pressure by 4%
- the reduction of total cholesterol by 6%
- A 47% reduction in levels of C-reactive protein, an inflammatory factor linked to cardiovascular disease. The two-year trial did not produce expected metabolic changes, but influenced other life span markers.[72]

A 23-year study by the National Institute on Aging (NIA) in Baltimore found that rhesus monkeys fed a diet containing 25-30% fewer calories did not live longer than rhesus monkeys fed a moderate calorie diet of healthy meals. However, the former group of monkeys did show lower rates of cancer, again supporting the idea that a lower calorie diet could help cancer patients.[73] Note: The food in the NIA's study had a natural ingredient base compared to purified diets containing a specific nutrient, mineral, or vitamin mix. Although natural-ingredient diets risk variation between batches, they are considered more complete compared to purified diets.

In a study involving mice to test how carbohydrate intake influences prostate cancer growth, despite consuming extra calories, all mice receiving low-carbohydrate diets weighed significantly less than those receiving a low-fat diet. In short, low-carbohydrate intake is an effective tool for weight maintenance. In addition, low-carbohydrate-consuming mice also had correspondingly lower fasting blood sugar levels.[74]

# Weight gain and cancer in women

Obesity has been linked to an increased incidence of hormone sensitive breast cancer. The majority of breast cancers in African American women are of this type.

The statistics for obese African American women and the incidence of cancer show a clear connection of rising values. As reported by the American Cancer Society, from 1999 to 2002, the obesity rate in black women was just 39 percent, but from 2009 to 2012, the obesity rate in black women rose to 58 percent. Meanwhile, the obesity rate among white women stabilized at about 33 percent. During the same period, the incidence of breast cancer steadily increased in black women, compared to stable rates in white women.

What might be the link between obesity and breast cancer? There might be several. First, obesity may alter the composition of collagen fibers such as those in the breast, which could then become cancerous. Second, excess body fat has been found to encourage cancer formation through higher levels of substances known as growth factors.

Third, the conversion of excess glucose into acetyl-CoA by the liver provides raw material to produce cholesterol to be used for the production of female hormones such as estrogen that promote cancer growth.

# An easy way to lose pounds if you have gained weight

No matter how careful we are, we all experience weight gain on many occasions during the year. This may occur from overeating now and then—such as at a party or during the holidays—or from drinking too many energy-containing (sugary) drinks, or even alcohol. Therefore, it is imperative to have a plan of action to deal with these times, preferably as soon as you detect it by noticing how much exactly you have gained above your "authentic weight"—the weight your intuition tells you is right for your body.

So whenever you feel a bit of weight gain, I recommend that, for the next few days, you switch to making your main meals consist of salads made with a variety of vegetables. Start with a mix of greens of your choice. Then add tomatoes, cucumbers, avocados, carrots, radishes, turnips, tender beetroots, bell peppers, both green and bulb onions, and other desirable items. Change the combination from one meal to the next. Be sure to make it crunchy. If you want, add nuts to the salads to increase the duration of your chewing.

Try to eat the salad without any dressing. The reason is to taste each nutrient without interference from any other flavor in the dressing. Using farm fresh, seasonal vegetables will give you the flavor as nature intended. I suggest that you avoid using items such as tomatoes that were selectively bred to increase sugar content.

If, after trying this method of eating, you find yourself getting hungry earlier than usual, go ahead and add a side dish of meat, fish, eggs or lentils to supplement your salad.

Above all, make sure you are not eating any grains or grain-flour products. An excess of glucose absorbed from grain-products will lead to insulin release that creates cravings for food, often more carbohydrate to satisfy the craving. When this happens, you fall into a cycle of eating at the mercy of your hormonal system, specifically, insulin. This is more than what your natural food intake control systems are designed for, leading to overeating followed by cravings followed by more overeating, *ad infinitum*. This leads to weight gain and, in addition, an excess of glucose that feeds your cancer cells.

# The reason you may gain weight quickly

The conscious part of your brain continuously seeks input. If not engaged, it will wander until it finds something interesting to concentrate upon. The subconscious mind, on the other hand, is always on autopilot. It keeps repeating what has been programmed, as often as it can so it can become as efficient as it can. The best example is the regulation of life-sustaining activities such as heartbeat, breathing, digestion, etc.

This interplay between your conscious brain and the subconscious mind is often the cause of overeating. Let's say you are at a social event, celebration, or even just a family meal. While the conscious part of the brain is occupied with talking, listening to a joke, celebrating, or paying attention to your boss, the subconscious mind, which has practiced the art of eating for many years, is happy to take over the act of food consumption for you. It smoothly guides you into nibbling on crackers and cheese, pushing chips into your mouth, buttering a roll, and eating the main meal while still talking and laughing. If you watch TV while eating, the subconscious mind is also at work, suggesting you have a second helping because your attention is focused on the screen rather than on listening to your brain tell you that you no longer need further nutrients.

The lack of conscious attention to eating is why so many people tend to gain weight so easily. Add to that the widespread availability of affordable foods, accessibility to a variety of artfully displayed dishes, and an abundance of munchies and desserts made with grain-flour, and it is clear that our culture makes it very easy to gain weight.

When we are young, we can reduce our weight by various methods, including increased physical activity. However, as we get older, it may take 3, 4, or more days to lose two pounds of added weight, even if we increase the intensity and duration of exercising. The reason is that while you may expend 250 or more calories during an activity, losing just two pounds of fat requires burning over 7,000 calories, making it nearly impossible to lose that weight without some type of plan.

In my view, the best way to do this is to re-activate the natural food intake regulatory system you had during your toddler years, when you ate only what you wanted and when you wanted. This method of eating is still archived in your adult brain. This nutrient intake regulatory system developed in humans through thousands of years of evolution and enables us to take in beneficial nutrients at just the amounts needed. Paying close attention to our senses of taste and smell is thus our evolutionary natural way to eat enough of what our body needs, without overeating.

# The best way to lose weight: Listen to your brain to avoid overeating

I believe that all creatures have a nutrient-intake regulatory system that was developed over the course of hundreds of thousands of years of our evolution. The evolutionary process created a chemical sensitivity in cells throughout the body that causes signals to be sent to the brain registering what nutrients they need. This capability to detect and respond to the chemical nature of a molecule is what enables all living organisms to take in beneficial nutrients and avoid harmful ones.

From the first days of a baby's eating food from nature (not mother's milk), the brain begins learning which foods provide which beneficial nutrients the cells in the body need. Every consumption of food leads to its digestion and the absorption of those nutrients. At first, the entry of these nutrients may be strictly transient actions, with little rationale. But as food consumption proves beneficial to the cell, the brain correlates which foods provide which nutrients. When the body needs those nutrients, the brain calls for us to repeat eating that food.

In this way, frequent use of the same food becomes identified with the nutrients contained in it. Thus, the brain learns the nutritional content of each food and prompts you to consume it when nutrients from that food are lacking in the body.

As we go from infant to toddler to youth to teenager and adult, whenever cells in the body need some beneficial nutrients, they send that signal to the brain. When enough of these signals are received, the brain creates the overall sensation of hunger. If you listen closely enough, the brain even directs you towards selecting particular foods by reminding you of how enjoyable they were to eat the last time. I submit that this is what guides you to desire certain items of food at various times of the day.

## CURIOUS TIDBITS

In a study involving twenty healthy men, a very low carbohydrate diet consumed for six weeks resulted in a significant decrease in body weight despite encouragement to consume more food to maintain weight. The investigators concluded that the higher satiety value of fat and protein resulted in significant reduction in voluntary dietary energy intake. Even more interesting was the finding that the entire loss in body weight was from fat. There was no change in their exercise pattern.[75]

# How your brain knows what you eat

While our cells are wired to our brain, signaling whenever they need nutrients, our evolution also resulted in developing receptors for taste and smell as part of our intake regulatory system. When we eat, the taste and smell receptors in the mouth and nose tell the brain what nutrients are being ingested. Chewing breaks food up into molecules that fit into the taste receptors and waft up into the smell receptors. They then send a signal to the brain indicating the nutrients that are in the food. Then as you eat, the brain, after comparing the quantity of nutrients from that food to the need, tells you whether you should continue eating or stop. The same comparison allows the brain to help you decide what you should choose to eat when you are offered multiple items, to get nutrients still needed in the body.

The proof of this notion is evident if you watch what happens when a baby is breastfed, versus one that is bottle-fed. During breastfeeding, the baby decides entirely alone when to stop sucking based on sensory signals generated by the release of milk into the baby's mouth. This is a built-in, natural regulatory mechanism in animals and humans. However, during bottle-feeding, not only is the rate of release different, the caregiver can coax the baby to take in more than the baby may need. The result is greater weight gain by bottle-fed babies compared to breastfed babies.

If you think about this evolutionary history of humans, "eating healthy" thus has a real, not vague, meaning. By paying close attention to your brain, you can "listen" for the signals telling you what to eat and how much of it, based on what your cells have told the brain about nutrients they need, not on the fullness of your stomach, or claims about the supposed nutritional value of a product.

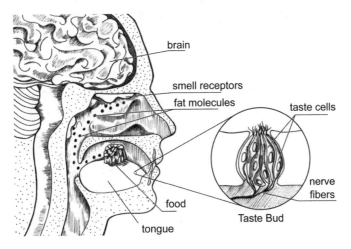

When we eat, the taste and smell receptors in the mouth and nose tell the brain what nutrients are being ingested. They send a signal to the brain indicating the nutrients in the food. After comparing the quantity of nutrients eaten, the brain tells you whether you should continue or stop eating. So chew slowly and listen to your brain's messages to avoid overeating.

# To avoid gaining weight, chew slowly and eat mindfully

By eating "mindfully," meaning slowly and focused on chewing the food in your mouth, you can learn how to stop overeating and, in the process, lose weight.

The act of eating slowly consists of three different stages.

- First, you experience the qualities of the food in your mouth by taking time to chew it and enjoy the taste.
- Second, you decide whether the food is appealing after enjoying each bite.
- Third, you swallow the food and decide whether to take another bite or stop.

Don't eat any foods that do not require chewing. Avoid blended, pureed, and liquid foods, for example, even if the proponents claim that they are tasty and you can easily get so many nutrients in that fashion. The basis for my objection to eating foods that do not require chewing is that this makes quantity control arbitrary based on how much is made, served, or is in a container, especially if you feel compelled not to waste food.

The same caution should be exercised when it comes to the consumption of fruits and vegetables. Chew whole fruits even if you have to cut them into pieces when you want to eat fruit. Do not drink fruit juices or blend fruits and vegetables into a smooth consistency to slurp them, for the same reason related to quantity control cited above.

In addition, when you eat, focus on the enjoyment of the experience. Don't watch TV or get distracted by talking through the entire meal. External activities that you do while eating can cause you to resort to "automatic eating," taking bite after bite and eating quickly such that you fail to pay attention to the various flavors in the food. When you do this, you are again not giving your brain enough time to register the nutrients, which helps you know when to stop eating.

# The importance of chewing

One of the differences between animals and humans with regard to food intake is that, for us, eating is more than just getting food into our mouths. The most noticeable difference is the cutting and cooking that no other animal does, nor did our ancient ancestors.

In fact, it is calculated that if modern humans had to chew raw meat along with natural roots, fruits, and vegetables, as our ancestors were forced to do before discovering cooking, it would take many hours a day of eating to get the nutrients needed for an adult. This extensive amount of time required to obtain one's nutrition, coupled with the difficulty of obtaining it, would have limited the free time available for other activities.

With improvements in agriculture and technology, it is obvious that humans were able to reduce the amount of time needed to eat to survive. Spending less time to get needed nutrients allowed more opportunities for all the advances in art, science, literature, music, athletics, and social interaction that have contributed to our cultural evolution.

Chewing is an important part of your brain's nutrient monitoring because deliberate, slow chewing allows the release of nutrients from each food item, at a speed that allows your brain to detect them in the mouth. If you want to better regulate your nutrient consumption during a meal in response to your sensation of hunger, the nutrient release in your mouth has to happen in a slow enough way that the concentration and the type of nutrient going down the throat can be monitored by your taste and smell receptors.

While water-soluble nutrients are detected by taste buds, volatile molecules released in the mouth during chewing waft up the nose to the smell receptors and alert the brain to the presence of nutrients on the way. Even the mechanical movements of your facial muscles activate the brain's monitoring system of nutrient intake. In short, all our systems are ready made for metering the amounts of nutrients entering the body. The combined sensory signals generated during a meal inform the brain of the nature and amount of nutrients about to enter the body, while creating an enjoyable experience.

To listen to and respect your brain's signals about hunger and satiation, you must learn to change the way you eat your meals. Chew each bite as thoroughly as possible. This act allows you to savor the natural taste and experience the differences in taste and the intensity of taste of each item. Eating fast, such as when you eat in a hurry for whatever reason, or swallowing foods that do not require chewing such as blended and pureed foods, is not conducive to your brain's need for the sensory organs in your mouth and nose to monitor your nutrient intake.

## CURIOUS TIDBITS

Cooking started about 1 million years ago, based on archeological evidence, and is credited with the reduction in tooth size and chewing muscles in modern humans compared to that of our possible ancestors, australopithecines. On the other hand, consider what could happen to the size of teeth and the facial muscles in future generations of humans if we continue our current trend of consuming more and more blended and pureed foods.

# Pay attention to your brain's hunger and satiation signals

At present, there is a lot of conflicting information about how and what to eat to remain healthy. For example, the US Dietary Guidelines Advisory Committee recently lifted its former recommendations that consumption of dietary cholesterol should be restricted. Some people may conclude that this is a license to eat as much animal protein, fat, and eggs as you wish. Meanwhile, other experts insist that a plant-based diet low in animal protein, harmful fats, and refined carbohydrates is best for you. They recommend a diet mostly of vegetables, fruits, whole grains, legumes, fish oil or flax oil, seeds and nuts for healthy living. Which is correct?

In my view, neither is completely correct, because they miss the point. The debate about diet incorrectly starts with the assumption that the sensation of hunger occurs when the body needs food for *energy*. This is wrong, because just one pound of stored fat represents 3,500 calories of stored energy, so anyone with the slightest amount of excess fat actually has plenty of stored energy.

I contend that the hunger sensation is generated when the brain, being the command center of our nutritional regulatory system, detects that key *nutrients*, not energy, will soon be lacking in the body's cells. The brain is continuously monitoring your body's nutrients and is already aware of the nature and quantity of any current nutrient deficiency when you feel the sensation of hunger. This is why even diabetics, who already have high blood sugar that represents energy, still feel hunger—they need certain nutrients.

Just as the brain detects an insufficiency of water in bodily fluids and generates the sensation of thirst, it signals hunger when it detects that needed nutrients are about to fall below optimum levels. This explains why you can feel the sensation of hunger at unpredictable intervals of time, even within a short time after eating if not enough of some key nutrients have been consumed. After generating the sensation of hunger, your brain effectively guides you towards what food to eat—and then monitors incoming nutrients by using your sense organs of smell and taste.

This means that rubrics like "eat a balanced diet," based on a calculated average using scientific studies, or "eat in moderation" are vague, unworkable recommendations. The same is true of consuming a fixed number of portions of recommended foods, as portion sizes can vary in restaurants and at home. And as you probably know, calorie counts have nothing to do with feeling satiated after eating. Ultimately, I believe that your best option is to pay attention to the messages you receive from your brain about when to stop eating. When the food no longer tastes as good as the first bite, your brain is sending you a signal that you have consumed most of the nutrients you need at that time.

# You need a variety of foods to get the nutrients your body needs

All living cells must carry out routine maintenance activities to survive and perform the task they are assigned. To manufacture the specialized products they need, each cell requires a specific set of raw materials, or nutrients. But one can't possibly consume all the nutrients the body needs for all cells to function properly, in each and every meal. It takes a wide variety of foods over many meals to fulfill the body's needs.

For example, calcium is needed for bone cells, and bone marrow needs iron and vitamins to create various blood cells. Brain cells need a continuous supply of glucose for their normal energy production, whereas muscle cells can use either glucose or fatty acids for energy, as you have learned.

Scientists do not yet know the exact number of nutrients the body needs, or whether some nutrients perform multiple functions, or whether different combinations of nutrients can accomplish the same functions as other combinations of nutrients. Since food supplies differ throughout the world, it would seem logical that the human body can successfully adapt to whatever nutrients are available to it. For example, in extreme cold climates where carbohydrate-containing foods are not as readily available, the native population has adapted by having a liver that manufactures glucose using amino acids derived from proteins or glycerol released from the fats they eat. As a result, peoples like the Inuit are perfectly able to maintain the level of glucose needed for neurons in the brain just as much as people who live amidst bountiful grains.

No one knows with certainty how much of each of these nutrients your body actually needs or how you get them from the foods you eat. That is why I suggest that eating a wide variety of foods is the best way to ensure you will likely ingest as many of these nutrients as possible. Inability to consume needed nutrients in a timely fashion could lead to improper functioning of immune system mechanisms and cancer formation.

Finally, pay attention to any cravings you have. They are literally messages from your brain indicating the lack of a specific nutrient needed at that time. However, avoid excess intake by chewing deliberately and paying attention to the reduction in your enjoyment of the food. Also, remain aware of the presence of energy-containing nutrients in the food items you crave.

# Be careful: Missing nutrients may cause you to overeat

Each food item you eat contains both *macro-* and *micro*nutrients existing in different combinations and ratios. Macronutrients are the larger energy-containing elements such as carbohydrate, proteins, and fats. Micronutrients are those needed in small quantities but nevertheless important in cell metabolism. Calcium, sodium, chloride, magnesium, potassium, phosphorus, and sulfur are considered macrominerals because they are required in large quantities compared to other minerals.

An inadequate intake of a nutrient needed at the time can lead to conditions that interfere with optimal utilization of another nutrient in the body.

Various foods, of course, contain differing amounts of those macro- and micronutrients. In adults, any time essential nutrients are available only in minute quantities embedded in foods that contain a lot of energy nutrients, the body may be forced to eat an excess of the energy nutrients just to get adequate amounts of the essential ones.

For instance, let's say you had a dish made of mixed nuts and only macadamias contain a micronutrient your body needs. You can't selectively pick out the macadamias. To get enough of the nutrient in the macadamias, you might have to eat five teaspoons of the mix containing all the nuts. The result of this is that the body must sometimes store the excess energy nutrients that are not used to produce energy at the immediate time.

The repeated intake of energy nutrients in excess of immediate need causes the body to increase its capability of storing energy nutrients. In short, you may be eating too much food just to be sure you are getting enough of the other nutrients from those foods. This overeating leads to fat storage and thus weight gain.

Worse: overconsumption can end up feeding cancer cells.

## CURIOUS TIDBITS

A class of medications called *thiazolidinediones* to treat Type 2 diabetes works by creating more fat cells to store glucose converted to fat, reducing blood sugar level. However, some of these medications, such as Pioglitazone, had to be removed from the market because of increased incidences of cancer. The reason: the signal from fat cells to prompt more stem cells to become fat cells also triggers cancer cells to multiply. (See the Special Section on Grains for details on how this happens.)

# Don't bother measuring nutrients

Science has identified 118 nutrients that are used at some point in human health. I suggest that the nutrients discovered to be useful to humans can be classified into three groups:

- water-soluble nutrients—these are detected when they come in contact with your taste buds.
- fat-associated nutrients—these waft up the back of the throat during a meal and stimulate smell receptors that inform the brain as to their precise nature.
- essential fatty acids—these are detected by receptors on the tongue.

When you eat, the combination of signals from these three groups, along with the mouth feel, is what you sense as the flavor of a food.

Nutritional science does not yet have the tools to understand or study the long-term health impact of any food containing multiple nutrients. Projecting nutritional values of the foods that a given individual consumes is complicated by the specifics of the circumstances, such as the combination of foods eaten during a meal, since the metabolism of one nutritional element could impact the absorption and utilization of another.

I therefore recommend that rather than trying to measure nutrient intake, you simply need to listen closely to your brain, which is helping you interpret the taste of the food as a signal to eat more or stop eating. As you consume foods, the receptors register the intake of the various nutrients and transmit signals to the brain, which produces the pleasure you experience when you are chewing the food. As you eat more of the item, you will find that your enjoyment of eating it will decrease; this is a signal from the brain that you no longer need the nutrients in that food. For example, when it comes to sweet-tasting foods, experiencing too much sweetness may produce the sensation of aversion; it's a signal that you have consumed too much sugar at one time. Perhaps this has happened to you if you ever ate too much chocolate or a sweet cake.

# Exercise is good for general health and possibly to fight your cancer

Whether you have been diagnosed with cancer or not, you should exercise. Physical activity is vital to the body, starting from childhood. The primary objective of exercise is to condition the lungs, heart, and muscles, regardless of your body weight. Conditioning develops reserve capacity available for use when you need it or when you become sick.

For example, an older person who does not exercise may have the capacity to deliver one liter of oxygen per minute to the tissues and a reserve capacity of three to four liters per minute. An athletically fit old person may have twice that much reserve. When an athletically fit older person develops a condition such as pneumonia, he or she has more available respiratory reserves. The same is true of a conditioned heart in an athletic older individual—it can pump more blood with less effort than an unconditioned person and has the reserves to help that person through a serious illness.

Similar reserves can be expected for the actions of other organs and systems in the body of someone who exercises. For example, conditioning allows your muscles to work longer before your brain senses the stress of exercise and makes you feel tired, compared to the brain that is not conditioned to exercising muscles. The ability of the human body to cope with unexpected events can be improved if your reserve capacities are maintained. Additional benefits of exercise come from improved blood circulation that helps the brain think more creatively and the skin to have a better tone. In addition, exercise helps keep blood vessels open and combats the major peripheral vasculature/neuropathy problem in diabetics.

In general, the evidence shows that you can decrease your risk of heart disease, hypertension, and diabetes, by adding an exercise regimen to your life. The American Cancer Society recommends physical activity of at least 150 minutes of moderate or 75 minutes of vigorous activity per week, because it can lower the risk of colon, breast, and endometrial cancer.

How might exercise help reduce your risks of cancer? One answer has to do with how your body uses glucose for energy when at rest and when exercising. During much of the day, muscles depend not on glucose but on fatty acids for their energy, the principal reason being that the normal *resting muscle* membrane is only slightly permeable to glucose, except when insulin is outside. But between meals, the amount of insulin secreted is too small to promote significant amounts of glucose entry into muscle cells. During exercise, however, muscles allow glucose to enter the cell without help from insulin.[76] The benefit of exercise is thus that it reduces the availability of glucose molecules to cancer cells. Exercise also lowers levels of hormones such as insulin and estrogen that contribute to cancer formation.

# The metabolic background of exercising

As explained before, the energy needed for metabolic activity is ATP, which cells produce in voluminous amounts on an ongoing basis. The supply of ATP in a cell is similar to having ready cash that can be used to complete a purchase.

As you may recall from earlier in the book, muscles sustain maximum power for about 10 seconds using readily available ATP. Then muscles turn on facilities that can instantly produce more ATP by splitting glucose molecules through the process of glycolysis outside the mitochondrion. The advantage of this is that ATP can be produced 2.5 times as rapidly as the production of ATP inside the mitochondrion.

However, at that point, inside the mitochondria, derivatives of fatty acids, amino acids, and glucose begin degradation by combining with oxygen to produce tremendous amounts of ATP through an extremely efficient process similar to that used by green leaves during photosynthesis. This energy is what powers the muscle cell after those first seconds.

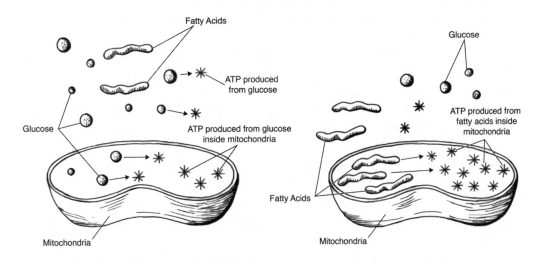

At the start of exercise ATP produced from glucose provides a burst of energy.

After about 10 seconds, ATP produced from fatty acids inside mitochondria provide continued energy.

During the first seconds of every physical activity, most of the energy is derived from glucose. But as you continue the activity, fatty acids in the mitochondria provide almost 80% of the energy to continue the activity. This means that it is not necessary to sustain a physical activity to achieve glucose reduction to starve cancer cells, as even exercising for small periods of time as often as you can will be of benefit.

# Why exercise is not useful for weight control in the long term

Weight control is a significant element in cancer prevention because your weight is a reflection of your food consumption. If you consume too much, especially grain-based carbohydrates that produce excessive amounts of glucose, you risk not only gaining weight, but also feeding cancer cells with their primary fuel, glucose.

In almost every book on weight management, exercise is usually mentioned as the key to losing weight and keeping it off. On the surface, you would think this makes sense. When you exercise, your muscles send a message to the brain for additional fuel. The brain sends another message to fat cells to release more fatty acids that can be burned as fuel. As the fat cells empty, you lose weight.

Many people, especially those young in age, do lose weight through exercising. While the body metabolism may increase about 100 percent during an extremely high fever, it increases more than 2,000 percent above normal during a marathon race.

However, I suggest not depending on exercise as your primary method to maintain body weight, for a variety of reasons.

First, most people simply do not exercise consistently enough to accomplish the goal of emptying their fat cells and maintaining lower body weight. Exercising burns very few calories relative to one's daily intake, especially if you are already overeating.

Exercise also tends to make people feel hungrier. You go out for a walk, a bike ride, or to the gym and you often return home and eat even more. So you might end up gaining weight rather than losing it.

Another problem with exercise is that it does not have the same impact on weight loss as you age. It is very difficult to keep up the level of activity needed to maintain a negative calorie intake when you have aging muscles. What used to take 20 minutes to burn 300 calories now takes 40 minutes or even an hour, as there is a gradual decrease in the ability to maintain skeletal muscle function and mass.

Given these reasons, I don't advocate exercise as a tool to lose weight because I believe exercise is neither necessary for weight management nor the best methodology to follow for it. Exercise is invaluable for one's health, but not a primary tool for weight management.

# Why exercise is not the way to lose weight

It is commonly accepted that exercise can help you burn calories and thus lose weight. But if you look closely at the numbers, you will see that this is not so, except for perhaps super-athletes who may exercise strenuously for hours per day. For a normal person, however, reliance on exercise for losing weight is not a realistic option, in the long term.

A woman weighing 140 pounds may expend 270 calories by walking 3.5 miles in one hour, 390 calories by riding a bike for one hour and going a distance of 10 to 12 miles, or 430 calories by running 30 minutes at a speed of 7.5 mph. But if she is doing one of these forms of exercise only two or three times per week, all the while consuming 1800 or 2000 calories per day, she will hardly make a dent in depleting her fat cells and losing weight. The same goes for men, although the numbers are slightly different.

Yes, you could get better results from exercising more and on a daily basis. On the other hand, the inability to exercise due to lack of time, facilities, or feeling tired often becomes an excuse for gaining weight.

Some professionals encourage exercise for weight control, claiming that the resting metabolic rate stays elevated after stopping exercise, which helps expend more energy. It is true that there is a gradual decrease in the resting metabolic rate after early adulthood and you can increase it with exercise. However, if the amount of energy expended on the actual exercise doesn't make a significant difference in your weight, the after-effects will be even less.

# Why exercise might help to reverse or halt your cancer

Currently, cancer experts recommend physical activity because it can lower levels of some hormones that contribute to cancer formation. In addition to supporting this, I add the following reason for you to find time to exercise.

First, a previous essay already mentioned that exercise might deprive cancer cells of their preferred fuel—glucose. So if your objective is to starve cancer cells of glucose, multiple episodes of exercise lasting for only a few minutes at a time can be used to accomplish that, because muscles generate energy primarily from glucose in the early stages of an activity.

But exercise also helps increase body temperature, and it's possible that elevating body temperature through a sauna or hot tub may also drive more glucose into normal cells to use, thus detracting from the amount of glucose that cancer cells can grab. However, this is yet to be verified. The sustained elevation of body temperature you get from exercise also improves the immune system and defense mechanisms of the body.

Exercise also increases oxygenation of tumor cells. This is valuable because, as explained, lower oxygen levels tend to promote conditions that benefit the spread of cancer, so it helps to increase your oxygenation. Increased oxygenation also enhances the effectiveness of drug- and radiation-induced cell death.

An expert panel of the International Agency for Research on Cancer of the World Health Organization estimated a 20% to 40% decrease in the risk of developing breast cancer among the most physically active women, regardless of menopausal status.[73]

A recent study indicated that the healthiest form of exercise that leads to life longevity is walking one hour per day. But any intentional movement of muscles, especially those of large muscles, can be considered an exercise. Your exercise can be done at home as part of routine housework or outside in your yard or garden. It can be done as part of specific work with a tool or as repetitions using equipment.

A regular exercise regimen—including walking, running, or resistance training—can keep your bones stronger and prevent osteoporosis. If your objective is muscle conditioning, prolonged sustained physical activity is what you need to do on a regular basis. Resistance training will add muscle mass, leading to better conditioning as well as increased energy expenditure during workouts.

For many people, the addition of exercise in their daily routines also reduces stress and offers the key to greater psychological happiness and wellbeing. Exercising in the company of others can help to build supportive relationships.

# The benefits of exercise in surviving cancer

No significant association has been detected between physical activity before diagnosis of breast cancer and survival. However, women who performed an equivalent of walking 3 to 5 hours per week at an average pace experienced reduced risk of death after breast cancer diagnosis.[74] In addition, women who exercised reported improved quality of life.

Although such statistics appear to quantify the duration of exercise relative to its health benefits, keep in mind that these recommendations are based on averaging the numbers of hours of exercise. This means there are some people who may have experienced greater benefits from less exercise than recommended, or vice versa. The bottom line is that you should do what you can. More importantly, do what you are comfortable with and for however long you are comfortable doing it. By choosing an exercise you like, walking rather than running for example, you are more likely to continue doing it. Gradually, you may feel the urge to push yourself to be more vigorous or devote more time to your exercising routine.

However, beware of certain types of activity. In short bursts of extreme muscular activity, for example a 100-meter sprint, as well as over long periods of intense muscular activity, oxygen cannot be carried to the muscles fast enough to oxidize the products of glucose breakdown. As a result, muscles use their stored glucose (glycogen) as fuel to generate energy. However, this leaves lactate as the end product, instead of the usual carbon dioxide and water when oxygen is available in sufficient quantities. The liver then converts lactate back to glucose, which cancer cells may benefit from. Therefore, you may want to stay away from this type of exercise.

Also, avoid strenuous exercise in low-oxygen conditions such as at high altitudes. While in ordinary cells, a low oxygen environment leads to increased production of reactive oxygen molecules that is toxic and results in cell death, cancer cells use the low oxygen condition to enhance their growth strategy. They do this by inducing the production of key enzymes involved in glycolysis. The same may be applicable to cancer cells experiencing low oxygen conditions in areas of the lung affected by an infection.

I suggest that you exercise in a fasting state, when your body tends to utilize fatty acids from your fat cells to provide fuel for energy generation in the mitochondria of muscle cells. Any release of stored glucose from the liver will be minimal. Meanwhile, since cancer cells do not have functional mitochondria, they are not able to produce energy using fatty acid as fuel, leaving them with little fuel.

# Environmental pollutants and inherited susceptibility

HUMANS ARE DIAGNOSED WITH OVER 100 TYPES OF CANCER. IN 1977, four scientists (Higginso, Muir, Doll and Peto) suggested that the majority of cancers are due to environmental factors and are therefore preventable. Inherited genetic conditions account for the rest. Some substances, such as naturally occurring asbestos and both naturally occurring and synthetic asbestos-like fibers (e.g., glass wool and rock wool), cause cancer through their physical rather than chemical effects. Other particulate materials that cause cancer include powdered metallic cobalt and nickel and crystalline silica. Usually, these agents produce cancer after years of exposure. In this section, we'll discuss how to avoid environmental pollutants and minimize your inherited risks.

# 10 tips to prevent cancer from environmental causes

1.  As much as possible, avoid any diagnostic radiation before age 30; it could increase breast cancer risk, especially for those who carry certain gene mutations.
2.  Cover your thyroid gland from radiation exposure during dental procedures.
3.  Avoid exposure to asbestos and other known causes of chronic inflammation.
4.  Avoid excessive exposure to UV radiation from the sun, especially if you have lighter skin pigmentation, by staying out of the sun between 10 a.m. and 4 p.m.
5.  Avoid cancer-causing agents in foods, even if a label says something like, "No carcino-genicity seen in animal studies at the concentration present," because the concentration and combination of many agents are unknown. For example, in a 2016 study by Portland State University, Oregon, researchers found high levels of pharmaceutical compounds such as painkillers and antibiotics, chemicals such as mercury and pesticides, and carcino-genic compounds in native oysters. The individual concentration of each such agent dis-covered was within safe levels outlined by state health officials, but the combined levels of all agents made for a toxic mix.
6.  Avoid using plastic containers to warm, bake, or cook food; having been made of chem-icals, these may release some of those chemicals into the food. If the food contains fat or oil that can trap the chemicals released, they may end up in your body. Similarly, don't use plastic containers inadvertently left in a hot environment, such as inside a car. Don't use a container or utensil, such as a cutting board, made of plastic for a long period of time as chemicals can be released from it into the beverage or food item due to degradation of the material used to make it.
7.  Be aware of exposure to chemicals such as nitrosamine, associated with gastric cancer, in skin products like lotions and creams, hair products for coloring and conditioning, latex products such as balloons, and in many food products and other consumables.
8.  Avoid any medication that can cause increased levels of cancer in a specific organ, if that medication is found to induce increased levels of a tumor marker in animal studies. Female sex hormones play a role in the development of breast cancer in women, and higher levels of testosterone are associated with higher levels of prostate cancer. Growth hormone may promote bone cancer.
9.  Alcohol, super-heated beverages, and sucking ice cubes raise the odds of cancer formation if cells that line the esophagus are damaged and cause your body to regenerate them too frequently. Accelerated regeneration risks gene mutations.
10. Avoiding cancer-causing agents is especially important during pregnancy because of faster cell division in the fetus. Toxin exposure in early life can later manifest itself as cancer due to changes to the gene controller called *epigene*. Based on the degree, duration, and timing of exposure, the type of cancer can change. Most fetuses experience 10 percent of tissue concentration of chemical agents of those in the mother.

# Recommendations on what to avoid if heredity is a factor for you

Given that many environmental factors can influence the development of cancer, if there is a hereditary factor in your family, it is important to avoid the following as much as possible:

- Exposure to unneeded chemicals in all forms, especially in processed foods you consume. You have no knowledge as to how completely that chemical will be detoxified in your liver, how it will interact with other chemicals in the body, whether it could have an additive effect at a site already responding to another trigger, or whether the concentration of the chemical fluctuates from one packet to the next during the manufacturing process.

- Keep in mind that the more food you consume away from home, the less control you have on intake of chemicals. Some chemicals may block response of cancer cells to chemotherapeutic agents.

- Exposure to the most easily avoidable triggers, such as infectious agents that are likely to induce cancer. Human papilloma virus, hepatitis B and C viruses, and Epstein-Barr virus have been identified as cancer causing. *Helicobacter pylori* are bacteria that both cause ulcers and increase the risk of cancer. Parasites that are associated with cancer include *Schistosoma haematobium* and the liver flukes. Any of these can interfere with cellular function and trigger cancer formation in susceptible individuals.

- A change in the number and type of beneficial gut bacteria, which has been found to be associated with the development of colorectal cancer. For example, persistent infection by clostridium is associated with chronic inflammation that can accelerate regeneration of cells in the colon and the potential for cancer formation.

- Consumption of antioxidants in high doses in an attempt to neutralize free radicals, as this may do more harm than good in certain types of cancer such as lung cancer among smokers. Talk with your doctor before taking antioxidant supplements.

# Stress, mindset, sleep, and hope

MILITARY METAPHORS SUCH AS "FIGHTING CANCER" AND "WAR ON cancer" have created a deep societal belief that cancer is a difficult and deadly disease that even with careful analysis, planning, and execution of treatment strategies has a potential for failure resulting in death, even though many diseases such as heart failure may have a worse prognosis than most cases of cancer. For example, the most common forms of cancer—non-melanoma skin cancers—are easily treated and almost always cured.

An important aspect of surviving cancer is to improve the quality of life by reducing any physical, emotional, and psychological distress. Be sure to use methods and/or substances proven to be effective, as this section will reveal.

# Managing your stress (Part 1)

When experiencing cancer, you may feel stress because of the uncertainties associated with the diagnosis and treatment. But it might also be because your brain cannot function well due to the lack of nutrients that cancer cells are confiscating for their own energy and multiplication. And of course, during your treatment, various drugs used for chemotherapy can affect your mood and create stress.

Managing your stress is a very important aspect of life in general, but especially after cancer. Feeling stressed releases growth hormone in the body, which causes increased production of glucose by the liver as well as the release of insulin from the pancreas. As we have discussed, both glucose and insulin aid the growth of cancer cells, with each one promoting a different aspect of multiplication. In addition, growth hormone causes the release of fatty acids from fat stores. Excess fatty acids in the blood promote muscles to switch fuel from burning glucose to burning fatty acids, thus leaving even more glucose in your bloodstream to feed cancer cells.

Although growth hormone lasts in the bloodstream for less than 20 minutes on average, it also causes the liver to manufacture small proteins called "insulin-like growth factors" that are similar to insulin in molecular structure. These proteins are normally produced by the activation of a gene called Igf2, and are a naturally occurring protein important for the growth of many cells in the body. These insulin-like growth factors released during stress can last in the body for 20 hours, on average. This greatly prolongs the growth-promoting effects of bursts of growth hormone secretion.

When all this is combined, it is clear that stress can create an internal environment in the body that makes it difficult to deal with challenges related to your condition and treatment. In addition, as explained, stress can trigger cancer cells that were not destroyed during the treatment to restart their multiplication process.

**⟦CURIOUS TIDBITS⟧**

The Pygmies of Africa have a congenital inability to synthesize significant amounts of insulin-like growth factor 1. This accounts for their small stature.

# The source and mechanism of stress

A wide variety of stimuli—anxiety, fear, pain, low blood sugar, starvation, etc.—can create stress in your life. When you are confronted with a stressful situation, you may have to take action—either fighting it or fleeing from it—almost immediately. The hormone that makes this possible is adrenaline, which raises the heartbeat and blood pressure and increases oxygen intake. Adrenaline causes release of glucose from the liver and ATP production through glycolysis. And, as you recall, glucose feeds cancer cells.

Cortisol is another hormone released during the stress response. Cortisol acts more slowly but in a more sustained manner to complement the actions triggered by adrenaline. Cortisol stimulates energy production from fatty acids and glucose production in the liver from glycerol released from fat molecules when fatty acids were separated. Cortisol also stimulates the breakdown of muscle proteins.

During extended periods of stress, the continued release of cortisol begins to cause damage to muscles and bone, and impairs hormonal and immune functions in the body. For example, changed patterns of serum cortisol levels have been seen in connection with abnormal levels of a hormone produced by the pituitary gland. Cortisol has been found to interfere with the proliferation of immune cells.

## Associated Stress

Forgive and forget is a common adage given to people experiencing stress. For some, forgiving may not be difficult, but forgetting can be. This is because their subconscious mind tries to associate a current event with similar events experienced in the past to help the conscious brain formulate a plan of action based on a full evaluation. The memory retrieval can link the current event to a similar stressful event, communication, or action, or it can be connected to a stressful past event with another person. People who are blessed with strong long-term memory are particularly susceptible to this and should make every effort to avoid dwelling on the past, lest it create stress disproportionate to the current event.

This biology clearly suggests that you must manage your stress if you have been diagnosed with cancer. Once you can accept it, carefully consider the available options to confront it and plan your future to overcome the challenge and lead a healthy life.

**CURIOUS TIDBITS**

If you are given cortisone as part of a medical treatment, it could result in the release of glucose from the liver to the extent of causing insulin release higher than what the body is used to. This, in turn, could generate the sensation of hunger because of low blood sugar, leading to increased food intake. Usually, this is a temporary situation that corrects itself when the cortisone therapy is terminated. This also means that experiencing a short period of excess insulin release need not make you susceptible to developing obesity and diabetes, as some have claimed in the past.

# Managing your stress (Part 2)

The activities of the human brain can be classified into three categories.

- At the *cognitive* level, we experience the input coming from our senses—vision, hearing, taste, smell, and touch.
- At the *intellectual* level, we analyze the input and reason it out.
- At the *emotional* level, usually based on the communications received from the intellectual level, the brain creates various feelings felt by human beings.

Under ordinary conditions, we deal with all of life's events in this orderly fashion. However, when you are under stress, the brain may shorten the intellectual/analytical part and create the emotional response to speed up the process. If you grew up in an environment dominated by physical or emotional stress, your brain may not have developed the faculties for orderly analysis of everyday stressful situations that everyone faces during life, from minor inconveniences to major medical problems such as cancer.

Since dealing with cancer requires you to be exposed to some amount of stress, let me recommend a new way to manage your stress. My suggestion will be to practice what I call "Detached Analysis." Start by thinking about a minor inconvenience you face. Now imagine it happening to someone you don't know. How would you analyze their situation? What would be your recommendations to them to deal with that situation? What would be your expectation of the results of his/her actions? How should the person respond if the result is not favorable?

Next, do a similar analysis with as many events in your own life as you can, imagining them occurring to someone else and using your analytical skills to solve the problems. Practice this type of thinking, and slowly it will become part of your thought process, leading you to actions based on a more orderly evaluation of any stressful situation you experience.

# Why people tend to eat when under stress

Adrenaline is released in the body in between meals to facilitate the use of fatty acids as fuel. If you become stressed when you're hungry, or vice versa, more adrenaline is released. One of the reasons eating helps you feel better is because food in your digestive system helps slow the release of adrenaline. Thus, the experience of feeling calmer and more relaxed after eating sets up a behavior pattern that promotes eating when you feel stressed.

A second reason people eat when feeling stressed is that the body's stress response causes you to seek out some action to mitigate the stressor. For many people, the action of preparing and eating helps them stop thinking about the stressor. With repetition, eating becomes an automatic reaction for how they meet the challenges of their lives.

Keep in mind that your stress-related behaviors, whatever they are and shaped by your social experiences, have been in place for a long time. They will take time to change even if you are highly motivated because of your condition. The first thing you need to do is to remove yourself from the environment that causes the stress, physically if possible. This will help reduce your exposure to the stress-causing stimuli. If that is not possible, try to indulge in another activity you enjoy doing, at least until neurons in charge of the stress response calm down to moderate the adrenaline release.

Another suggestion to reduce stress-related eating is to perform a physical activity, such as going for a quick walk, to make use of the adrenaline that is being released.

# Minimize negative frames of mind

In general, a negative frame of mind is a stressful environment. The longer you stay in a stressful environment, the greater the chance of continued growth of cancer cells. This means, in my opinion, it is a critical goal to conduct your life so as to not stay in a negative frame of mind. In fact, this may be easier than striving to cultivate a positive frame. Some ways to do this:

1. Never decline a chance to be with anyone who can express genuine pleasure. Such a person is the product of a loving, nurturing environment during the first few years of his/her life. That person's attitude will often cheer you up, if not inspire you.

2. If you have to be associated with someone who is insecure and fearful by nature, spend as little time as possible with that individual. The experience of stress in the pre-teen years, when one has to make decisions based on reasoning to become an independent individual, could create such an individual. While the person may show sympathy and concern for you, he or she is also likely to launch into talking about their fears and insecurities about you and everyone else who may have similar or related conditions as you have. Usually, such narratives do not bring on a feeling of happiness or well-being and will boost your level of stress.

3. Be prepared to cope with an abundance of sympathies from well-wishers, especially soon after your diagnosis. Look at the inner being of your friends and acquaintances and see only what you want to see, regardless of the qualities visible or expressed. For example, someone may invite you and expect you to accept the invitation to spend time with them, or to come over wanting to be with you with the expectation that they can help you cope with the situation. Acknowledge their desire to help, but accept only if you feel it is worth it.

4. Never deny yourself a chance to experience an enjoyable meal, when you are hungry. Of course, I am not suggesting gorging at each meal. Take your time to eat what you enjoy and, more importantly, chew and savor each bite of food you eat.

5. If someone offers to pray for you in a religious or communal setting, you have to decide whether the frequency of the activity and the number of people involved will create a repeating reminder of an experience you want to put behind you so you can move on. However, for some believers, knowing that others are praying on their behalf could be reassuring.

# Mind over cancer: Using mental exercises to defeat cancer

The thought of cancer recurrence can be overwhelming. If the thought process continues, fear and stress follow. The best way to prevent a fearful thought from returning is to replace it with another, less fearful, thought, shifting the focus so that you engage a different set of neurons.

Although there may be changes in your brain related to aging, most people maintain the brain's ability to create a thought in one part of the brain and direct it to another part to formulate a course of beneficial action. What I am suggesting is that, just as you can initiate a voluntary action based on your thought process, it may be possible to influence your body's automatic functions.

When combined with conventional medical care for cancer, repeated mental exercises such as imagining killer cells searching, attacking, and destroying cancer cells hiding in the body can be an effective way to feel in control of what is happening inside you. Keep in mind that you are not asking your brain to do anything new. Your body's killer cells are perfectly capable of destroying cancer cells at the command of the immune system. You are only consciously encouraging what the body is programmed to do naturally.

During standard cancer treatment, this exercise can improve the quality of your life by moderating some of the side effects, such as anxiety, depression, and pain.[75] However, even after a treatment is over, creative visualization can help people with cancer feel more positive.

In addition, a continued practice of silent visualization of seeking and destroying may keep the already-trained immune cells proactive by practicing their skills. More importantly, this may teach the newly minted immune cells returning from the gut after their general security briefing to become proficient in identifying the enemy and destroying it.

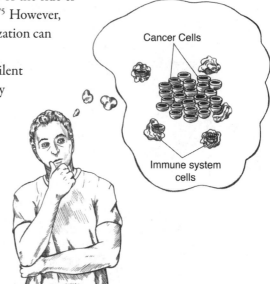

Imagine killer cells searching, attacking, and destroying cancer cells hiding in your body. You are not asking your brain to do anything new. You are only consciously encouraging what the body is programmed to do naturally.

# Get rest and good sleep

You spend almost one-third of your lifetime in sleep, physically unable to move, even for your own safety. When sleep overwhelms you, your brain will create signals, overriding all other desires.

During the 18th and 19th centuries, people used to sleep at least 9.5 hours per night. The average length of sleep today in the US stands at 6 hours. Sleep deprivation lasting for a long time can make you feel chronically tired and less efficient, especially with mental tasks.

Adequate sleep is vital to self-care after cancer. Animal studies show that disrupted sleep inhibits immune cells that stop cancer cells, while promoting cancer growth through blood vessel formation. Therefore, you have to plan your activities so that you get adequate rest both physically and mentally.

If your sleep is disturbed, find out whether it is related to changes in your tolerance for ambient conditions, such as temperature, due to your cancer or chemotherapy. If so, look for ways to adjust the temperature in your bedroom to accommodate your body's reactions. See if your sleep is being disturbed by other factors such as dry or itchy skin due to the side effects of medications. The intensity and type of light emitted by your television, computer, and other appliances may change the setting of your biological clock. Stress and anxiety can also be other factors.

Since the main objective of sleep is to give nerve cells a chance to do repair and maintenance work, involve your brain in challenging activities such as reading and doing puzzles during daytime, not just before bedtime. Avoid drinks with stimulants such as caffeine in the nighttime. Establish a routine with a specific time to go to sleep. Keep the room cool and uncover head and toes to dissipate any excess heat from the body.

Or, if you prefer, catch up on your sleep during the daytime with brief naps that will also calm your mind.

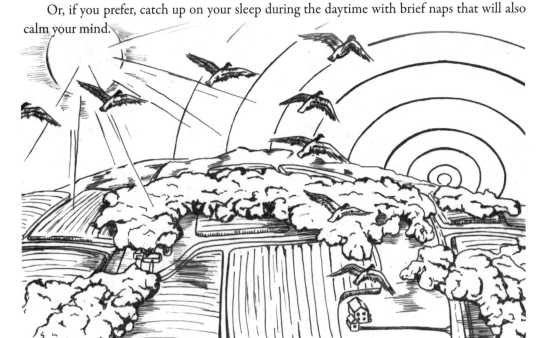

# The physiology of sleep

The timing of many physiological activities, including sleep, is programmed on 24-hour rhythm cycles called circadian rhythms. It is not surprising that about 10,000 neurons in charge of this mechanism are influenced by particles of light, because the existence of nearly all life on earth depends on light from the sun.

Specialized cells in the retina of the human eye respond to the short-wavelength light (450 nanometers) of the morning. This causes a reduction in melatonin production, leading to wakefulness. Electronic devices that emit light of similar wavelength may interfere with melatonin production, thus delaying the initiation of sleep.

Without exposure to light, the circadian rhythms of the body gradually go out of phase with the actual time of the day. However, even a brief 15-minute burst of bright light can reset the 24-hour circadian rhythm of biological activities.

The human biological clock, calibrated to daily light and perhaps temperature cycles, controls a wide range of physiological processes such as release of hormones, sleep-wake cycles, bowel movements, body temperature, and feeding patterns.

For a long time, it was believed that the purpose of sleep was to give muscles time to rest and recuperate. The brain was mostly inactive except for maintenance of the functions of vital organs. However, based on patterns of electrical activity, it was detected that the brain is still quite active, releasing signaling molecules that produce or inhibit sleep.

The reason behind the value of sleep and dreams has not been clearly understood. I propose that sleep is for nerve cells to repair and, above all, test all the networks between neurons after the required maintenance work, especially the ones that have been used the most during wakeful hours. Therefore, it is not how many hours of sleep you should have based on calculated averages from human studies, but how many hours of sleep it will take to complete the repair and maintenance work needed to keep cells and their connections in good working order. This, in an adult, as you can imagine, will depend on usage of nerve cells prior to going to sleep.

## CURIOUS TIDBITS

- Great frigate birds of the Galapagos Islands sometimes fly continuously over the ocean for up to 10 days with one side of their brain asleep.

- A dramatic exhibition of light-induced biological activity is the modification of a bird's behavior. Light-induced activation of vitamin B2-associated proteins of nerve cells in the bird's brain allows them to become receptive to magnetic waves from the earth. Light is thus how a bird's brain is able to chart the route for navigation to migratory destinations.

# Anticipate the happy events of life

I was diagnosed with cancer myself several years ago.* I experienced the same emotions I explained in this book for anyone diagnosed with cancer. I asked questions and, when I could not get answers that satisfied me, I started to develop explanations, ending in the creation of this book.

In addition, I decided that since I did not ask to be born, my primary objective in life should be to be happy without inconveniencing or hurting others striving to accomplish the same.[77] The past is in my memory and the future in my imagination. I am lucky that I have accomplished close to what I had imagined for myself because getting "close enough" is the practical way of life, in general. My life has been filled with a wide range of experiences, and for that, I am grateful.

Starting today, look at the rest of your life as an adventure journey towards a general destination that, like any other journey, will be modified based on the expectations you carry forth and the experiences you have. Treat people around you as if meeting them for the first time. Plan a project that you have always wanted to accomplish but never got time to do, or a new one you want to try. Feel good about your ability to do it. If the result is what you anticipated, feel satisfied. Do not, I repeat, do not wait for validation from another person or group to feel satisfaction about your accomplishment, for two reasons. First, instead of satisfaction, you may feel unhappiness if you don't get what you were expecting. Secondly, you may feel discouraged to start another project for fear of failure.

Every day concentrate on one pleasing thing or event you're going to enjoy that day or in the near future. It could be the shopping you are planning or visiting a friend or a relative. It could be the details of a trip you are about to take or the fruits you expect from your labor in your garden. The moment you start thinking about what will occur, you'll feel good. Even if you repeat this process many times, you'll still feel happy about the anticipated event. You have learned to enhance the enjoyment of a pleasing experience.

With practice, you can anticipate and enjoy more than one event at the same time. When the first real life event is about to be over, you can start shifting your attention to the next event, thus feeling less saddened about the end of one pleasing event because you're already thinking about the next one. You could store these events in your memory as a diary of future events. The first few pages can be filled with descriptions of happy events that are anticipated within the next few days; the middle pages can hold images of events in the near future; and on the final pages, you can sketch events expected to come later. The descriptions are removed as the events pass through reality or when they are found to be unattainable, and new ones are added and anticipated. In this way, you can stay busy and happy by looking forward to different categories of future events such as a book to read, a friend to visit, a project to be done, or a story to write.

---

* For those who are curious, my cancer was of the lymphatic system. I tolerated chemotherapy with minimal discomfort. I am in remission, under surveillance, practicing what is presented in this book as best as I can and enjoying life.

# Savoring pleasurable events

In my opinion, happiness is not simply the absence of unhappiness or stress. This is not to say that unhappiness and stress will not interfere with your sense of happiness, but to say that you should want to be happy, and be ready to take action to experience happiness.

There is a curious biological fact about happiness that is worth understanding. There are various molecules, such as endorphins and dopamine, released in your brain to produce a sense of satisfaction and enjoyment. By design, the effects of these are short-lived compared to the effects of molecules such as adrenaline and cortisol released in the body in response to stress or unhappy events. What this means is that you have to have stimuli, planned or unplanned, to force the release of neurochemicals in your brain if you want to experience happiness.

Look back at your life to remember the pleasant things that have happened. Think of your life as a snapshot of all your experiences. You feel good reminiscing. When you look through a photo album, you can recall incidents that still elicit happy memories. Now, train your mind to dwell on experiences before they happen and get more pleasure out of them. In other words, anticipate the pleasant things in life before they actually occur. The neurochemical releasing neurons do not know the difference between a current event, one in the memory, or one that has not happened yet.

When you are alone, appreciate the solitude, as it is the only way to experience the mystery of what life and living is all about. Develop a new awareness of who you are, and how unique you are compared to everyone around you. Like a word in a sentence, you complete the meaning of the existence of those who came before you and those who will follow. Imagine the world as you would like it to be—harmonious, loving, and peaceful. Call the exercise meditation, if you like, but keep the sensation of it for as long as you can experience it. If it helps, sit down comfortably, and listen to recorded music of your choice and stay there, lost in the melody.

Each time you step outside and encounter anything—a shrub, a tree, an animal, or another person—appreciate how each one is unique in its own way. Look deeply into a lovely flower. Take a moment to really appreciate the shape, color, curvature and arrangement of the petals. What caused the plant to put that flower in that particular place? How did the plant know what type of pigments and how much of them were needed by that flower? What caused the bud to open up not too soon but to wait for the petals to be ready? How did the flower know its pollen would attract a honeybee or its nectar would feed a hummingbird? Will the flower ever know how much it was appreciated?

To feel the fullness of life, you need to experience love that would immerse your body and soul in it. To create that love, you need to accomplish an objective. To accomplish an objective, you need a reason. Some people find the two, love and reason combined, in accomplishments achieved through a vocation or calling.

When you feel lonely, look at things around you and form an opinion. When you hear people talk, form an opinion. When you express your opinion to others, you get a response. You are not alone anymore. Ultimately, the love you get from others is one of the best experiences you cherish in your life.

# Find compassionate caregivers

I can't overemphasize the need to have a compassionate cancer care specialist and a team of caregivers on your side. Such a team should be in place and be there to help you right from the initial office visit. You will need help and support for so many things that no longer seem ordinary:

- receiving results of tests from the oncology staff
- reviewing your clinical progress or lack of it
- discussing medications to control side effects including allergic reactions
- reducing the dose of medications causing side effects in an orderly manner while keeping an eye on the benefits sought
- preventing your exposure to infective agents while you are extremely susceptible due to immune suppression
- defining your living environment and transportation needs

You may feel that you are at a point when you can no longer think or rationalize. Regardless of the type of cancer, you may be constantly wondering what the future holds for you. As your brain analyzes the signals and looks for a reason to anchor a sense of hope, fear can grip the whole mind, spiraling the thought process into a sense of hopelessness. You may experience these moments many times. Sometimes you may have to brush them aside and go through the next salvo of treatment and side effects overriding your own despair, simply for the sake of your loved ones.

Your caregivers at home, your family, your friends, and your work and play companions are all vital. Use them to every extent they offer you.

# Challenges of your support team

Once you are diagnosed with cancer, many thoughts and actions may seem to paralyze you, especially the fear of the unknown related to your prognosis, as well as the following:

- feelings of guilt based on what you could have done but did not do
- the impact of your condition on your family and loved ones
- the social stigma and disruption of participation in events that you have been part of
- the side effects of treatment
- the feeling of helplessness, especially when you have to ask for physical, intellectual, and emotional support

Cancer creates a multitude of feelings in you, in your family members, colleagues, friends, and even in strangers who happen to hear about it. This means that you may be surrounded by a number of people who are concerned and fearful about your condition. It also means, while these people can be a source of comfort, they can also be a source of anxiety because of their own worry about you. Some may even wonder aloud to you about their chances of getting cancer.

Friends and family may want to reassure you, some may want to give you material support, others will offer emotional support, and some may give you greeting cards or trinkets in an attempt to cheer you up.

While you can appreciate the intention behind each one of these actions, it can also remind you of your condition and create a new round of anxiety and stress each time you encounter the person or the memento, unless you put all this in perspective.

Talk to those from whom you truly want help and support. If some of them are not comfortable helping you because of their own insecurity, don't let that bother you. Keep the mementos away from your sight because chances are you want to get on with your life without being constantly reminded of your cancer.

# Living to 120 (yes, really!) while surviving cancer

Some of us would choose a path to live forever, if given a chance. This is understandable because, individually, every cell with a nucleus has the potential of infinite life, dividing time after time, inherited from the original cell. In this sense, the desire to go on forever is part of our genetic legacy. It is embedded within every organism, though it is a legacy that was sacrificed for the sake of a life of companionship and comfort when one of the ancestors of the cell decided on group living.

When cultured in a nutrient-rich favorable environment of a laboratory, cells lose the ability to survive after about 50 divisions. Cells taken from an older live human have been found to be capable of dividing, on an average, twenty more times.

Putting it all together, it appears to suggest that with proper care, one can extend the life of the average person to almost 120 years from a current average of about 80.

However, a longer life also means more mutations and more chance for cancer formation. Or mutations that may lessen the functional capabilities of your vital organs, so that you'd end up with other conditions and problems that degrade the quality of life or even endanger your life itself.

Each of us thus can only do our best to survive for the longest life with the least number of malfunctions in our cells. The key to this, in addition to the environment we live in and what we eat, is not to be in a hurry. For example, Greenland sharks can live upward of 500 years by moving through arctic waters at roughly one mile per hour and growing less than an inch per year.

Allow me to ask you a philosophical question. Suppose you die after leaving a cell from your body to a laboratory that keeps it alive in a culture. Will your soul stay with the still living portion of your being? (After all, it is believed that your soul started its journey on this earth in a single cell formed after two sex cells joined to form one.) What if the cell multiplies and some daughter cells are shipped to different laboratories? Where will your soul be?

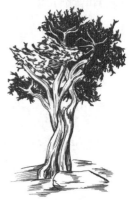

Bristlecone Pine Tree
3000–5000 Years old

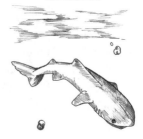

Greenland Sharks
500 Years old

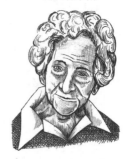

Jeanne Louise Calment
(1875–1997)
122 Years old

Some living things live for millennia or for centuries. It appears that human life can extend to more than 120 years. What is the secret?

# Evolution and longevity

The evolution of every living thing, as explained by Darwin, will always continue, albeit at a very slow pace. However, in an organism facing persistent environmental challenges, adaptive changes can happen more rapidly. Adaptations can be structural—such as changing the external shape or internal organization; or they can be behavioral—such as a sharpening of instincts or learning capacity; or they can be functional—such as improving the immune system, or harnessing the body's temperature regulation system. Some adaptations allow the organism to continue on, better suited to live in a particular environment. If the adaptive change favors survival, it could lead to genetic changes that are passed on to the next generation.

The evolution that has benefitted the human race most is cultural, caused by our sense of awareness. A life of experience and enjoyment by a human being is made possible through learning, memory, imagination, creativity, and reasoning, among other attributes. All these are manifestations of a brain with a permanency of nerve cells and longevity of connections between them, leading to conscious awareness.

If a human had to divide into two, like a one-celled organism does, to become immortal, nerve cells would have to be reborn and reestablish connections with other newborn nerve cells. This can completely change the personality of the individual in a way that you may as well be a different person altogether.

Nature has essentially gone this route by splitting genes and packing two half-sets in sex cells that join to become a new human being with the potential to live to an age when the process can be repeated, with the newly created pairs of genes carrying all the instructions needed for continuation of life. In this respect, every person is part of a lineage for propagation of the human race, similar to a single-celled organism passing the genes to the next generation.

If you are not happy with having only your genes immortal, but want to keep yourself living as long as possible, study the Bristlecone pine in California's White Mountains. They live for thousands of years due to slow and deliberate growth. Application of this principle to humans means slowing your metabolic activities to the minimum by avoiding stress and infections, and providing cells with needed nutrients in a timely manner.

In short, to live long: try to enjoy every moment; lead a slow, purposeful, and leisurely life; respond to stress in a deliberate, measured way; get regular exercise; create a happy family environment; enjoy friendly conversations; and eat a varied, primarily plant-based diet.

# Key Points and Conclusions

When you are diagnosed with cancer you experience a multitude of emotions, ultimately ending up with the sense that it is possible you will die from it. Some may accept this as their destiny, since everyone has to die one way or another. And as you have learned, formation of cancer cells is natural and therefore inevitable. So its prevention is unrealistic...but surviving it is possible. We know that since the progression of cancer does not follow a predictable course, there are modifiable factors that can influence your lifespan after the diagnosis. The strategy I have outlined to influence the progression of cancer does not include medications and their side effects, but has the potential of preventing dying from it. Why not try it?

## Summary of key points

This book has covered a good deal of ground and it can be confusing and overwhelming. However, I hope that you have learned a lot about how the body works, what cancer is, and what you can do to survive it. You have far more control over what you may have thought possible to prevent your cancer from spreading and to keep in check the cancer cells within you.

Working with your oncologist, you can take back control of your body—through knowledge of what is happening inside you, along with avoiding grains to starve cancer cells, with exercise to support a healthy body, with changes to your diet to build your immune system, and by dealing with stress and avoiding a negative frame of mind.

Here is a summary of the main points that this book has covered.

### The Adam Cell Theory

I propose that the urge to multiply is a fundamental and integral part of life itself. The ability of self-replication existed before the construction of an independent living cell, as we know it.

For example, viruses, more ancient than human organisms, are life forms made of very small bits of genes. Yet even they have the capacity to make copies of themselves using the resources of a host cell they inhabit, as we know very well from every viral epidemic, both in humans and animals.

My theory is that the most fundamental characteristic of cancer—the uncontrollable multiplication of cells—reflects an unchangeable biological fact. From the evolution of the very first functional cell that existed on earth, which I call the Adam Cell, the urge to multiply is built into the essence of our cells. No matter how dysfunctional or disabled a cell becomes, it will always, at a minimum, seek to replicate itself.

### Cancer cells are constantly forming

A fundamental fact of life is that our body is continually producing cancer cells. Most are destroyed by programmed self-death and by the immune system, or their mutations are repaired.

In general, some mutations are beneficial, as they serve as adaptations that ensure coping with their environment for continuation of life. The conditions in which the organism lives, the external environment, play a role in how the genetic capabilities are expressed and more importantly, evolve. So, the obvious question is: Are humans evolving in such a way that cancer, the result of mutations, endows humans with an evolutionary advantage? It is clear that cancer, depriving neighboring cells of their nutrients and ultimately causing the death of the organism, is not an advantageous evolution of the organism itself. But, by the same token, there might be an as-yet unknown evolutionary advantage because of mutations. We may not understand this advantage at this time.

### Requirements for cancer formation

Mutations do not necessarily lead to cancer. Three basic conditions have to be met for uncontrolled cell multiplication to occur. Imagine a train engine idling on a flat railway track. The train is like a normal cell with intact metabolic activities.

1. If someone releases the brakes, it does not automatically result in the train's movement. Similarly, *mutations*, even when they make the cell capable of multiplication, do not automatically result in uncontrolled divisions.

2. The gear has to be engaged for the engine to start moving, or the engine needs a push if it is in neutral. Similarly, *growth promoting agents*—such as insulin, insulin-like growth factor, estrogen or fat cell-released agents, and perhaps other yet to be identified stimuli—are needed to urge multiplication of a mutated cell.

3. Once it starts, the engine cannot keep going indefinitely if there is no fuel supply. Similarly, for the vast majority of cancer cells, multiplication will proceed only as long as glucose is available.

## The need to detect cancer ASAP

The first and best approach to cancer is to detect gene mutations before they reach the cancer threshold, especially in people who may have inherited susceptibility. However, there is still much to learn about detecting and dealing with cancer. Consider these questions:

- Which cell in the target organ or tissue should one look at to detect cancer? How often?

- Although cancer susceptibility is caused by gene mutations, predicting the effects of small genetic changes on cell division is very difficult. One could periodically look for a telltale sign such as a particular protein linked to a mutated gene or parts of mutated genes in samples collected from a person. But, how often one should have the test?

- If a signaling molecule is detected, how are we to know what effect it will have, not only on a target cell but also on other cells?

- If a particle of mutated gene is detected, should we take aggressive steps or take a more patient approach? This may depend on factors such as family history, for example.

- If we detect one type of cancer in an organ, should we stop looking or continue to rule out yet another one?

- What if cancer cells, originally sensitive, mutate during treatment and become resistant to the therapeutic agent? Keep in mind that the original cancer may have had cells mutated in different ways but not activated until after the start of the treatment.

- Is it possible to detect accelerated rate of multiplication of a particular cell line? Only future research will tell.

This is not to say that we should not gather information as to the percentage of people who may develop cancer in a particular geographic, dietary, behavioral, or demographic context. This kind of information can define a person's risk for certain types of cancer and help him or her be prepared to avoid or deal with it.

One area where the benefit of early detection of cancer is indisputable is in a young person who would like to have children, but who would likely be infertile if he/she survived cancer. Sperm banking is a viable option for men. For women, the options range from cryopreserved mature eggs, embryos created by in vitro fertilization, or preserving ovarian follicles that could later be stimulated to produce eggs.

## Methods that medicine has developed to fight cancer

Here is a review of the current and potential medical capabilities to deal with cancer cells. Your doctor may be using one or more of these, based on your genetic and cancer cell metabolic profile:

- Once we detect mutated cancer cells early, we can seek to remove them using surgery or other methods.

- We can silence an overactive gene by molecular slicing.

- We can destroy an offending gene by sending a designer peptide with an attached drug straight to the location.

- We have drugs that can directly inactivate mutated genes.

- We can disrupt signals from mutated genes for multiplication, or inhibition of immune cells. For example, growth and multiplication activities of a cell are controlled by "checkpoints" to ensure their stability and progression. Scientists can develop therapeutic interventions targeted at specific checkpoints inside cancer cells to prevent them from multiplying.

- We can block the formation of new blood vessels that help cancer growth.

- We can kill the cancer cells by blocking the exit of waste products from them.

- We can replace mutated genes with synthetic ones.

## Methods you have to fight cancer through your own actions

- Starve cancer cells; avoid eating grains and grain-flour products to reduce the amount of glucose in your bloodstream. Cut out breads, pasta, rice, corn, pizza, cakes, pies, doughnuts, and recipes that use grain-flour starch.

- Focus your meals on fresh vegetables, meat or fish, and substitute sweet potatoes, whole cooked potatoes with skin, and lentils in place of the grain-based carbohydrate you would have eaten.

- Spice up your dishes with fresh, natural spices such as thyme, oregano, basil, chili peppers, cumin, coriander, ginger, turmeric, black pepper, and others that improve your enjoyment of food and help you eat less.

- Pay attention to the signals from your brain about hunger and satiation. The moment when food no longer provides enjoyment in your mouth is a signal from your brain to stop eating. Don't wait for your belly to be full to end your meal, as this is a sign of overconsumption.

- Eat mindfully. Chew your food slowly, enjoying each bite and savoring the ingredients and the flavors. Add nuts of your choice to increase the duration of chewing. On the other hand, don't eat any food that does not require chewing. Avoid blended, pureed, and liquid foods.

- Reconnect with your authentic weight and lose body fat, which is associated with increased cancer risk.

- Exercise not to lose weight but to help starve cancer cells and boost your immune system. Exercise with others for support.

- During a period of stress, react deliberately after analysis of known facts.

- Sleep when your brain tells you, for as long as it needs to do repair and maintenance.

## The concept of curing cancer

Curing cancer, one of the major public and private objectives for decades, has proven elusive, not because we don't know the mechanism of cancer formation, but because we don't know how to selectively stop the mutations that permit it. Living in an environment that is constantly changing, some mutation of genes is necessary for our survival. The causes that lead to mutations, the speed with which they occur, the order of activation of enzymes, the availability of nutrients to form a new cell including a new nucleus, and interference during the process of multiplication—all these determine whether the result of mutation is beneficial or not.

Since every cell in our body (except red blood cells) has genes that could be mutated by various external and internal mechanisms, from my perspective, every one of us technically lives in a pre-cancer state. We all need to be vigilant because the world around us will cause every person to be exposed to chemical agents, particulate material, biological molecules such as viruses, and energy sources that can enter our body through the nose, mouth, skin, etc. that might lead to gene mutations, especially after prolonged exposure. Over time, there is an unavoidable and almost continuous production of free radicals due to metabolic activities inside cells. All these can react with proteins, including the DNA inside your cells, causing genetic mutations. And as we age, the chance for mutations leading to cancer increases.

The idea of curing cancer marches on, however, as our knowledge keeps changing. But for each step forward, we sometimes take one (or two) backwards. It seems frequent today that the results from some studies may suggest one causative factor or method of treatment, which later is found non-consequential after another study. Anxiety created by the first report, spread widely through the media, may not subside with the publication of the new study, either because the new information did not reach everyone or some are skeptical of the results.

It is expected that most of the above limitations and inconveniences can be overcome in the near future by targeted immune therapy. However, even this approach may not slow the expected increase in the *incidence* of cancer in many parts of the world, creating significant physical, emotional, and financial challenges for the world.

Considering that cancer cells do not need a special environment to start the process, everyone is at risk for developing cancer and most people do generate cancer cells in their body, only to be destroyed by their own surveillance mechanisms. But unfortunately, the longer we live, the higher our odds of getting cancer. At the present state of our knowledge, hoping for a cure for cancer is akin to hoping that we can cure old age. In fact, one could ask why are we not seeing more cancers given the number of mutations that a person experiences during a lifetime.

My suspicion is that with all the mutations experienced, many cells that could become cancerous may not have the ability to reactivate the archived information to multiply like an embryonic cell, even if the external environment is conducive to multiplication. This is similar to animals losing some of their abilities to survive in their native habitat after being kept in captivity for years.

## "Curing cancer" is not actually possible... at least for now

Although the ability to screen, detect, classify, and offer targeted and personalized cancer treatment strategies has improved over the years, the term "cure" is applicable only if we are speaking about stopping a cancer that has established itself. Medicine is indeed getting better at "curing" some existing cancers in the sense that they can sometimes be removed or stopped.

However, we have no guarantee that even when we can't detect any remaining cancer at the original site, some cancer cells aren't hiding in another part of the body, waiting to multiply when the conditions are right. In addition, since cancer cells can appear in the body at random, a "cure" may not last for long.

Finally, despite our hope, the concept of "curing cancer" does not at this time mean that science knows how to prevent cancer from occurring in the first place. There is no vaccine that prevents all cancers from happening in an individual in the way that we have vaccines that can completely prevent polio, smallpox, measles, and other illnesses.

## Immunization to prevent cancer

One achievable goal we are able to accomplish is to better promote cancer prevention related to viral infections through immunizations. For example, the HPV immunization could be used more widely, and HBV vaccine is cancer-preventive. In fact, the prevention of viral infection-induced cancer is a more attainable goal compared to that of curing cancer. We need more vaccine research related to viral-induced cancers, because, in effect, we have no real way to permanently stop cells from mutating in the wrong ways and then replicating themselves over and over again. That is their innate drive.

This means that our strategies for "curing" cancer are *ad hoc*; we are only able to stop a few types of cancer, one at a time. And the cure for one type of cancer may not be effective in another. In fact, even in the same organ, breast for example, two different types of cells such as ones that line the milk duct and others that line the milk-producing lobule, could experience totally different mutations when subjected to the same cancer-causing environment. These two types of cells exhibit different types of cancer, and while one responds to one therapeutic agent, the other could be resistant to the same agent.

Moreover, each cancer could develop more complex and different biomolecules, making it difficult to use the same strategy to screen, detect, classify, and treat the same type of cancer in another person. This predicament with cancer is no different than what we experience with each new epidemic of influenza that arises from a new virus created by mutation, making it difficult to control using the vaccine made from the previous year's viruses.

## Preventing cancer-related death is the most important priority

Nature, having created life and endowed it with the capacity to replicate, must have foreseen the possibility that every cell has the urge to keep multiplying. As explained earlier, nature has put controls in place to regulate the start and termination of cells multiplying forever. Nature also prescribed cell multiplication to be done in an orderly fashion during normal cell regeneration activities in any cell line.

However, this feat of nature is clearly not foolproof. We see these mistakes in the abnormal growth of tissue, called polyps, in the small and large intestine, stomach, nose, sinuses, urinary bladder, and uterus. These are most often inconvenient, not deadly. And even when these cause serious inconveniences, such as blocking a passage like the nose, they are considered benign, based on the almost normal architecture of their constituent cells.

But since mutations and adaptations are necessary for continuation of life, nature also expects the formation of occasional cancer cells as inevitable. It appears that nature has made provisions to stop the process, or at least make it difficult to continue when a cell gets the urge to multiply uncontrollably, resulting in metastasis and its various consequences. Perhaps this is nature's reason for creating the capability and willingness for self-destruction called apoptosis and giving immune cells a chance to mount a programmed attack to eliminate unruly cells.

## Hope for you

For a person with cancer, the mind often tries and tries to associate the diagnosis with every conceivable causative factor that he or she may have encountered. What starts as an attempt to identify the causal factor(s) could become an obsession to avoid every agent known to trigger cancer formation, however small it might be. Thinking that you are at a much higher risk of dying from cancer than you actually are could lead to living a life of caution, fear, and hopelessness. In fact, some people, especially men, fearing the possibility of a diagnosis of cancer, avoid having the necessary checkups needed for routine maintenance of the body.

What I am proposing in this book is that you must learn to work with nature by not interfering with mutations that may have to happen for the benefit of human survival. We therefore need to find ways to allow our natural immune system to be on guard and strong by providing needed nutrients in a timely fashion, and not tax the system unnecessarily by getting infections and risking environmental exposures that could be avoided. This means doing everything you can to avoid toxins and carcinogenic agents, exercise regularly, sleep well, learn to minimize your response to stress, and enjoy life as best as you can.

However, the primary emphasis of this book is about making sure that you eat healthy. By that I mean to consume the nutrients your body needs while avoiding what it doesn't. Keep in mind that plants, animals, and humans are all part of a natural world because nature provided nutrients for their sustenance. Kittens, cubs, and toddlers know exactly what and how much they want to eat, and it is the same as what they need.

Cancer cells that survived the natural elimination process in the body need an energy source before they can embark on the destructive path of metastasizing. What I have explained in this book is how to attack cancer's vulnerability by reducing the level of glucose circulating in your blood. This will also help you reduce the level of insulin in response to your lower blood sugar level, and that further dampens the speed of cancer cell multiplication and movement.

Be conscious of your feelings at all times. Try to enjoy each of your daily activities to the fullest. Choose activities you want to take to achieve your objectives.

You now have the knowledge of why cancer starts and how it survives. Armed with this understanding, you can plan the strategy to navigate around the iceberg in you—your cancer.

# Notes

1. Indian Express, Oct 2016.
2. Cree, L.M., Samuels, D.C., et al. (2008). "A reduction of mitochondrial DNA molecules during embryogenesis explains the rapid segregation of genotypes". *Nature Genetics*. **40** (2): 249–254.
3. Knudson A G (1971): Mutation and Cancer: Statistical Study of Retinoblastoma. Proc Natl Acad of Sci. USA. **68**:820-823
4. Törnroth-Horsefield, S.; Neutze, R. (2008). "Opening and closing the metabolite gate". *Proc. Natl. Acad. Sci. USA*. **105** (50): 19565–19566.
5. Lichenstein P, Holm NV, et al: (2000). Environmental and Heritable factors in the causation of cancer. The N. Engl J Med. **343**:78-85
6. Sorensen TIA, Nielsen GG, et al: (1988). Genetic and environmental influences on premature death in adult adoptees, N Engl J Med **318**:727-32.
7. Tumor Suppressor Genes, edited by Yue Cheng, ISBN 978-953-307-879-3, 344 pages, Publisher: InTech, Chapters published February 03, 2012 under CC BY 3.0 license DOI: 10.5772/1337
8. Nogueira L, Foerster C, et al: (2015). "Association of aflatoxin with gallbladder cancer in chile." *JAMA*. **313** (20): 2075–2077
9. Shay, JW; Bacchetti, S (1997). "A survey of telomerase activity in human cancer". *Eur. J. Cancer*. **33**: 787–91.
10. Fine EJ, Miller A, Quadros EV, Sequeira JM, Feinman RD: Acetoacetate reduces growth and ATP concentration in cancer cell lines which over-express uncoupling protein 2. Cancer Cell international 2009, 9:14:11.
11. Schwartz M: (1961). A biomathematical approach to clinical tumor growth. *Cancer*, **14**:1272-1294. And Fine et al. Same as #10
12. Kim JW, Dang CV (September 2006). "Cancer's molecular sweet tooth and the Warburg effect". *Cancer Research*. **66**: 8927–30.
13. Kim, R., Emi, M., and Tanabe, K. (2007). Cancer immunoediting from immune surveillance to immune escape. Immunology *121*, 1–14.
14. Teng, M.W.L., Swann, J.B., et al. (2008). Immune-mediated dormancy: an equilibrium with cancer. J. Leukoc. Biol. *84*, 988–993.
15. Ho VW, Leung K, et al. (2011). A Low Carbohydrate, High Protein Diet Slows Tumor Growth and Prevents Cancer Initiation. Cancer Res 71:4484-4493.
16. Peto, R., Roe FJ, et al. (1975). Cancer and aging in mice and men. *British Journal of Cancer* 32:411–426.
17. Kuper H, Adami HO, Trichopoulos D. (2000). Infections as a major preventable cause of human cancer. J Intern Med **248**:171-183
18. Coussens LM and Werb Z. (2002). Inflammation and cancer. *Nature*. **420**: 860–867.
19. Abegglen LM, Caulin AF et al. (2015) Potential mechanisms for Cancer Resistance in Elephants and Comparative Cellular response to DNA Damage in Humans. Jama.com
20. Onitilo AA, Engel JM, et al. (2012). Diabetes and cancer I: risk, survival, and implications for screening. Cancer Causes Control 23:967-81.
21. Wen W, Shu XO, et al. (2009). Dietary carbohydrates, fiber, and breast cancer risk in Chinese women. Am J Clin Nutr **89**:283-289.
22. Thompson, Di Angelantonio, Gao, Sarwar. (2011). Diabetes Mellitus, Fasting Glucose, and Risk of Cause-specific Death. N Engl Med **364**:829-41
23. Masur K, Vetter C, et al. (2011) Diabetogenic glucose and insulin concentrations modulate transcriptome and protein levels involved in tumour cell migration, adhesion and proliferation. British Journal of Cancer. **104**:345-352.
24. Ryu TY, J ParkJ, Scherer PE. (2014). Hyperglycemia as a Risk Factor for Cancer Progression. Diabetes Metab J. **38**:330-336

25. Schwartz M et al. Same as #11

26. Jacob T., Agarwal A., et al., (2016) Ultrasensitive proteomic quantitation of cellular signaling by digitalized nanoparticle-protein counting. Nature.com/scientificreports. June 6:28163

27. Kantoff PW, Higano CS, et al. (2010) "Sipuleucel-T immunotherapy for castration-resistant prostate cancer" *N. Engl. J. Med.* **363** (5): 411–22

28. Seidel UJ, Schlegel P, Lang P (2013). "Natural killer cell mediated antibody-dependent cellular cytotoxicity in tumor immunotherapy with therapeutic antibodies". *Frontiers in Immunology.* **4**: 76.

29. Pettersson, A; Richiardi L .et al. ( 2007). "Age at Surgery for Undescended Testis and Risk of Testicular Cancer". *NEJM.* **356** :1835–41.]

30. Ho et al. Same as #15

31. Lehninger Principles of Biochemistry. Sixth Edition, D L Nelson and M M Cox editors. W H Freeman and Company, N Y 2013

32. Jadvar H., Pinski JK, Conti PS. (2003). FDG PET in suspected recurrent and metastatic prostate cancer. Oncology Reports, **10**:1485-1488

33. Stattin P, Bjor O, et al. (2007) Prospective study of hyperglycemia and cancer risk. Diabetes Care, **30**: 561–567

34. Augustin LS, Dal Maso L, et al. (2001): Dietary glycemic index and glycemic load, and breast cancer risk: a case-control study. Ann Oncol **12**:1533-1538.

35. Derr RL, Ye X, et al. (2009): Association between hyperglycemia and survival in patients with newly diagnosed glioblastoma. J Clin Oncol **27**:1082-1086.

36. Augustin et al. Same as #34.

37. Lee C, Lizzia Raffaghello L, et al. Fasting Cycles Retard Growth of Tumors and Sensitize a Range of Cancer Cell Types to Chemotherapy. *Science Translational Medicine* 08 Feb 2012:

38. Moulton CJ, Valentine RJ, et al. A high protein moderate carbohydrate diet fed at discrete meals reduces early progression of N-methyl-N-nitrosourea-induced breast tumorigenesis in rats. Nutr Metab (Lond) 2010, 7:1

39. Ho et al. Same as #15.

40. Pavlova NN, Thompson CB. The Emerging Hallmarks of Cancer. Cell Metabolism (2016), **23**;27-47.

41. Park J, Sarode VR, et al. (2012). Neuregulin 1-HER axis as a key mediator of hyperglycemic memory effects in breast cancer. Proc Natl Acad Sci U S A **109**:21058-63.

42. Dong C, Yuan T, et al. (2013). Loss of FBP1 by Snail-mediated repression provides metabolic advantages in basal-like breast cancer. Cancer Cell. **23**:316-31.

43. Vaughn AE, Deshmukh M. (2008). Glucose metabolism inhibits apoptosis in neurons and cancer cells by redox inactivation of cytochrome c. Nat Cell Biol **10**:1477-83.

44. Waterhouse C, Jeanpretre N, Keilson J: (1979). Gluconeogenesis from alanine in patients with progressive malignant disease. Cancer Res **39**:1968-1972.

45. Thompson, Di Angelantonio, Gao, Sarwar. (2011). Diabetes Mellitus, Fasting Glucose, and Risk of Cause-specific Death N Engl Med **364**:829-41

46. RJ Klement and U Kammerer, (2011). Is there a role for carbohydrate restriction in the treatment and prevention of cancer? Nutrition & Metabolism **8**:75

47. Levin I: (1910). Cancer among the American Indians and its bearing upon the ethnological distribution of the disease. J Cancer Res Clin Oncol **9**:422-435.

48. Rodin J, Slochower J. (1976) Externality in the Nonobese: Effects of Environmental Responsiveness on Weight. Journal of Personality and Social Psychology. **33**;338-344

49. Goodwin. J, Neugent ML, Lee S. Y., et. Al. The distinct metabolic phenotype of lung squamous cell carcinoma defines selective vulnerability to glycolytic inhibition. *Nature Communications* **8**, Article number: 15503, Published online 26 May 2017

50. Lee J. V., Carrer A., Shah S., et al. Akt-Dependent Metabolic Reprogramming Regulates Tumor Cell Histone Acetylation, Cell Metabolism Published Online: July 03, 2014

51. Rodin J. (1985) Insulin Levels, Hunger, and Food Intake: An example of Feedback Loops in Body Weight Regulation. Health Psychology; **4**;1-24

52. Melkonian S. C., Daniel. C.R., Ye. Y., et.al. Glycemic Index, Glycemic Load, and Lung Cancer Risk in Non-Hispanic Whites. Cancer Epidemiology, Biomarkers & Prevention. March 2016

53. Fine et al. Same as #10.

54. Irhimeh MR, Fitton JH, Lowenthal RM (2007). "Fucoidan ingestion increases the expression of CXCR4 on human CD34+ cells". *Exp Hematol.* **35**: 989–94.

55. Kazłowski B; Chiu YH; et al. (August 2012). "Prevention of Japanese encephalitis virus infections by low-degree-polymerisation sulfated saccharides from *Gracilaria* sp. and *Monostroma nitidum.*" *Food Chem.* **133** (3): 866–74.

56. Oba K, Teramukai S, Kobayashi M, Matsui T, Kodera Y, Sakamoto J (June 2007). "Efficacy of adjuvant immunochemotherapy with polysaccharide K for patients with curative resections of gastric cancer". *Cancer Immunology, Immunotherapy.* **56** (6): 905–11.

57. Kazłowski et al. Same as #55.

58. Fine et al. Same as #10.

59. Rich AJ and Wright PD. (1979). Ketosis and Nitrogen Excretion in Undernourished Surgical Patients. J. Parent Enteral Nutr **3**:350-354]

60. Maurer GD, Brucker DP, et al. (2011). Differential utilization of ketone bodies by neurons and glioma cell lines: a rationale for ketogenic diet as experimental glioma therapy. BMC Cancer **11**:315.

61. Maurer et al. Same as #60.

62. Ericson U, Sonestedt E et al. (2007). High folate intake is associated with lower breast cancer incidence in postmenopausal women in the Malmö Diet and Cancer cohort1´2´3 Am J Clin Nutr **86**; 434-443

63. Sung B, Prasad S, Yadav VR, Aggarwal BB (2012) Cancer cell signaling pathways targeted by spice-derived nutraceuticals. Nutr Cancer **64**:173-197

64. Kaefer CM, Milner JA (2008). The Role of Herbs and Spices in Cancer Prevention. J Nutr Biochem **19**:347-361

65. Grivennikov, S., Karin, E., et al. (2009). IL-6 and Stat3 are required for survival of intestinal epithelial cells and development of colitis-associated cancer. Cancer Cell **15**, 103–113.

66. Hutchins AM, Brown BD et al. (2013) Daily flaxseed consumption improves glycemic control in obese men and women with prediabetes. Nutr Res **33**:367-375

67. Park Y, Subar AF, Hollenbeck A, Schatzkin A (2011). "Dietary fiber intake and mortality in the NIH-AARP Diet and Health Study." *Arch Intern Med.* **171**: 1061–8

68. LoConte NK, Brewster AM, et al. (2017). Alcohol and Cancer: A Statement of the American Society of Clinical Oncology. J. Clin Oncol. Published online, November 7, 2017.

69. Bianchini F, Kaaks R, Vainio H (2002) Overweight, obesity, and cancer risk. Lancet Oncol **3**: 565–574

70. Stattin et al. Same as #33.

71. Snnivasan SR, Myers L, Berenson GS (1999). Temporal association between obesity and hypennsulinemia in children, adolescents, and young adults The Bogalusa Heart Study Metabolism **48** 928-34

72. September, 2015 issue of *Journal of Gerontology: Medical Sciences.*

73. The National Institute on Aging (NIA) at the National Institutes of Health. August 29, 2012 online issue of *Nature.*

74. Masko EM, Thomas JA, et al. (2010) Low-Carbohydrate Diets and Prostate Cancer: How Low is "Low Enough"? Cancer Prev Res (Phila). **3**:1124-1131

75. Volek JS, Sharman MJ, et al. (2002). Body composition and hormonal responses to a carbohydrate-restricted diet. Metabolism. **51**:864–70

76. Guyton and Hall: Textbook of Medical Physiology Twelfth Edition. Saunders Elsevier Philadelphia, PA 2011

77. Bianchini et al. Same as #69.

78. Holmes MD, Chen Wy, et al. (2005) Physical Activity and Survival After Breast Cancer Diagnosis, *JAMA.* **293**: 2479-2486.

79. Roffe L, Schmidt K, Ernst E (2005). "A systematic review of guided imagery as an adjuvant cancer therapy." *Psychooncology* (Systematic review). **14**: 607–17

# Glossary

**acetyl CoA** A molecule that participates in many chemical reactions involving amino acids, fatty acids, and glucose inside cells

**Adam Cell** In my theory, this cell represents an original ancestor of all cells that multiply. Codified into in its genes is the ability to divide into two whenever it needed to survive

**adiponectin** a hormone released from fat cells

**adjuvants** a substance or agent that is capable of boosting a biological or chemical reaction

**alpha-fetoprotein** a protein found in human fetus

**amylase** the enzyme that digests complex carbohydrates

**apoptosis** the natural process of self destruction when cells are not functioning correctly or have mutations

**ATP** *adenosine triphosphate* (ATP) the energy carrier cells use to power their functions

**Australopithecines** possible human ancestors

**authentic weight** the weight your body is most comfortable at and which allows your blood sugar and triglyceride levels to stay in a normal range

**bifidobacterium** the most common bacterial variety that survives and thrives in breastfed infants

**biosurgery** a process involving introduction of live organisms such as bacteria into a solid tumor to destroy it

**BMI (Body Mass Index)** a measure of proper body weight correcting for differences in height

**butyrate** a fatty acid compound that provides nourishment for the cells lining the colon

**Cancer Genome Atlas** a project to catalogue genetic mutations responsible for cancer

**cancer promoter** a chemical or agent that helps cancer cells

**checkpoint** regulatory center inside a cell to ensure proper status for entry from one metabolic phase to another

**committed stem cells** stem cells specialized with characteristics consistent with various tissues such as muscles or nerves

**DNA** a molecule that carries the genetic instructions used in the growth, development, and functions of all living organisms

**embryonic stem cell** undifferentiated cells from the embryo that can change into specialized cells and divide to produce more cells of any type in the body

**epidemiological studies** A continuous, systematic collection, analysis, and interpretation of data to identify risk factors for disease and targets for preventive healthcare

**fatty acid burn switch** muscle cells switch to burning small fatty acid compounds between meals when blood glucose is low. In diabetes, because of high circulating levels of fatty acid, this occurs on a consistent basis, creating the conditions for high blood sugar and diabetes

**gene manipulation** the process of altering genes to reverse the mutations that adversely affect its function

**glucose transporters** mobile units that pick up glucose molecules from the cell membrane and bring them in for the cell to use. Humans have at least 12 types of glucose transporters

**glycogen** glucose that is stored inside cells. The liver holds about 120 grams of glycogen to be released as glucose when blood sugar level is lowered

**glycolysis** the process of converting glucose molecule to generate ATP

**growth activating genes** a pair of genes responsible for initiating cell multiplication

**growth inhibiting genes** a pair of genes responsible for telling the cell to stop multiplying

**hepatitis B vaccine (HBV)** a vaccine that prevents hepatitis B

**ketone bodies** these (acetoacetate and 3 hydroxybuterate) are produced in the liver from fatty acids. Muscle cells can burn ketone bodies, allowing your body to function without eating grains

**malignant melanoma** cancer that develops from the pigment-containing cells

**mature fully differentiated cells** cells with an assigned function in an organ or tissue

**microRNA** messengers made of Ribonucleic acids that carry instructions from genes inside the nucleus to the workers in the cell

**mitochondrion** factories where a cell produces a lot of its energy in the form of ATP

**mutation** codification of any change, for good or bad, to the genes in a cell

**natural killer cells (NK cells)** a special group of cells with the ability to detect and destroy cells that are dysfunctional

**nucleotide** organic molecule that is used to build DNA and RNA

**oligosaccharide** a form carbohydrate containing three to ten molecules of simple sugar found in breast milk and plants

**organelles** small units within cells that perform specific tasks

**PET scan** a nuclear medicine functional imaging

**photodynamic therapy** a form of phototherapy involving light and a chemical substance to elicit cell death

**Pioglitazone** a drug of the thiazolidinedione class

**proton beam therapy** a form of cancer therapy using proton beams

**resistant starch** a form of starch that escapes from digestion in the small intestine of healthy individuals

**RNA** ribonucleic acid, essential for various biological coding, decoding and expression of genes

**single-nucleotide polymorphism** variation in a single nucleotide

**telomerase** an enzyme programmed to add length to telomeres

**telomeres** protective caps on chromosomes to prevent them from deterioration or fusing with each other

**triglycerides** the main constituents of body fat in humans and other animals

**tumor suppressor gene** a gene that prevents uncontrolled multiplication of a cell

**umami** savory taste that forms one of the five basic tastes together with sweetness, sourness, bitterness, and saltiness

**vascular endothelial growth factor (VEGF)** a protein that stimulates the formation of blood vessels

# Index

# Acknowledgments

As with any major project, many have helped me in this book.

I owe special thanks to M.V. Pillai. M.D., FACP, Clinical Professor of Oncology, Thomas Jefferson University, Philadelphia, and Dr. Kay Bauman for their review and suggestions

I thank Dr. George Kannarkat, Dr. Antony Poothullil, Dr. Venugopal Menon, Dr. Cliff and Delann DeBenedetti, Julie Blume, Paul and Alice Thoppil, and Paul Nelson for their friendship and support.

I want to thank Tim Kummerow for his beautiful illustrations on the front and back cover that convey my concept that cancer is like an iceberg and we must learn to sail around it.

I thank Kayla Benson for her adept drawings that help make the ideas in the pages more understandable and enjoyable to read.

I thank Ryan Scheife for his thoughtful book and cover design.

Thanks to Julie Simpson for her copyediting and proofing.

Finally, I thank my editor and publisher, Rick Benzel, for his commitment and extensive guidance in helping me develop my writing and transform my manuscript into this important book.

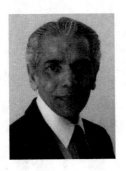

# ABOUT THE AUTHOR

**John M. Poothullil, MD, FRCP** practiced medicine as a pediatrician and allergist for more than 30 years, with 27 of those years in the state of Texas. He received his medical degree from the University of Kerala, India in 1968, after which he completed two years of medical residency in Washington, D.C., and Phoenix, Arizona and two years of fellowship, one in Milwaukee, Wisconsin and the other in Ontario, Canada. He began his practice in 1974 and retired in 2008. He holds certifications from the American Board of Pediatrics, The American Board of Allergy & Immunology, and the Canadian Board of Pediatrics.

During his medical practice, John became interested in understanding the causes of and interconnections between hunger, satiation, and weight gain. His interest turned into a passion and a multi-decade personal study and research project that led him to read many medical journal articles, medical textbooks, and other scholarly works in biology, biochemistry, physiology, endocrinology, and cellular metabolic functions. This eventually guided Dr. Poothullil to investigate the theory of insulin resistance as it relates to diabetes. Recognizing that this theory was illogical, he spent several years rethinking the biology behind high blood sugar and developed the fatty acid burn theory as the real cause of diabetes.

His study of diabetes also led Dr. Poothullil to further research the link between diabetes and cancer. While working on this book, he was himself diagnosed with cancer of the lymphatic system. Following chemotherapy, he is in remission, under surveillance, practicing what he presents in this book and enjoying life.

Dr. Poothullil has written articles on hunger and satiation, weight loss, diabetes, and the senses of taste and smell. His articles have been published in medical journals such as *Physiology and Behavior, Neuroscience and Biobehavioral Reviews, Journal of Women's Health, Journal of Applied Research, Nutrition,* and *Nutritional Neuroscience.* His work has been quoted in *Woman's Day, Fitness, Red Book* and *Woman's World.*

Please visit DrJohnOnHealth.com to follow Dr. Poothullil's blog and to send us your questions and feedback on how this book has changed your life.

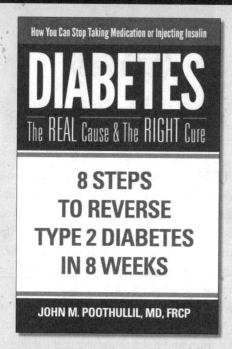

*Award Finalist in the "Health: Diet & Exercise" category of the 2017 Best Book Awards*

Unless YOU do something about it, your diabetes will be a progressive disease because medication and insulin injections do not reverse it. This book provides NEW INSIGHT that will lower blood sugar and halt your diabetes. Based on twenty years studying the scientific research on diabetes, Dr. Poothullil shows that the theory of insulin resistance cannot be valid. The REAL cause of diabetes is the consumption of grains and grain products. The RIGHT cure for diabetes is not medication or insulin injections, but altering your diet.

## Warning

Insulin injections and insulin-releasing medications make no sense if you are supposedly insulin resistant. In fact, these are endangering you:

- Insulin makes you hungry so you eat more and gain weight, making your diabetes worse
- Insulin injections lower blood sugar, but they do not prevent diabetic complications— damage to nerve cells, blindness, kidney failure, and atherosclerosis—and could cause abnormally low blood sugar which could be life-threatening
- Insulin promotes cancer cell growth, which is why there is a higher incidence of cancer among people with diabetes than those without

Don't risk having Type 2 diabetes for the rest of your life, regardless of your age or how long you have had it. Learn how to reverse diabetes using 8 simple steps in 8 weeks so you can restore your health.

ISBN: 978-09984850-0-3 | NEW INSIGHTS PRESS

# FOR MORE INFORMATION
## about Preventing Type 2 Diabetes

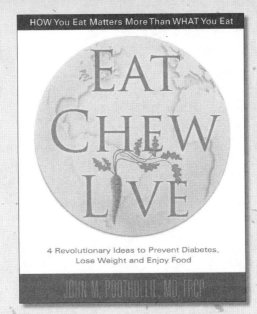

HOW You Eat Matters More Than WHAT You Eat

EAT CHEW LIVE

4 Revolutionary Ideas to Prevent Diabetes, Lose Weight and Enjoy Food

JOHN M. POOTHULLIL, MD, FRCP

*Selected as Winner in the Nutrition Category in the Beverly Hills Book Awards*

*Eat, Chew, Live* introduces a new science-based theory on the cause of obesity, high blood sugar, and diabetes. Discover how you can shed pounds and lower your blood sugar in a simple, natural way, without medications. No programs to follow, menus to cook, or products to buy.

*Eat, Chew, Live* will motivate you to reconnect with your authentic weight, listen to your body's hunger signals, and learn to eat mindfully.

You, a family member, or your friends may have high blood sugar (prediabetes) or diabetes and not even know it—making this book worthwhile for everyone.

*Eat, Chew, Live* teaches you how to avoid high blood sugar. With insight and inspiration, Dr. Poothullil shows you how to:

- lower blood sugar
- enjoy food without overeating
- lose pounds and keep them off
- see your relationship with food in a new light
- reconnect with your body's "authentic weight"
- get off of diabetes medications or insulin injections.

"A fascinating inquisition into the metabolic machinery of the human body with common sense advice on diabetes prevention."

—Sumit Bhagra, MD, FACE, Endocrinologist, Mayo Clinic Health System

ISBN: 978-0-9907924-0-6 | OVER AND ABOVE PRESS